Music and Creativity in Healthcare Settings

Through a series of vivid case studies, *Music and Creativity in Healthcare Settings: Does Music Matter?* documents the ways in which music brings humanity to sterile healthcare spaces, and its significance for people dealing with major illness. It also considers the notion of the arts as a vessel to explore humanitarian questions surrounding serious illness, namely what it is to be human. Overarching themes include taking control; security and safety; listening; the normalisation of the environment; being an individual; expressing emotion; transcendence and hope and expressing the inexpressible.

With an emphasis on service user narratives, chapters are enriched with examples of good practice using music in healthcare. Furthermore, a focus on aesthetic deprivation contributes to debates on the intrinsic and instrumental value of music and the arts in modern society. This concise study will be a valuable source of inspiration for care givers and service users in the health sector; it will also appeal to scholars and researchers in the areas of Music Medicine, Music Therapy, and the Medical Humanities.

Hilary Moss, PhD, MBA, is Senior Lecturer in Music Therapy at the University of Limerick, Ireland, and formerly Director of the National Centre for Arts and Health, Dublin. For more on her work see UL Talks: www.youtube.com/watch?v=j1t3lr_eWwI.

Music and Creativity in Healthcare Settings

Does Music Matter?

Hilary Moss

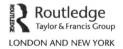

Routledge
Taylor & Francis Group

LONDON AND NEW YORK

First published 2021
by Routledge
2 Park Square, Milton Park, Abingdon, Oxon OX14 4RN

and by Routledge
52 Vanderbilt Avenue, New York, NY 10017

Routledge is an imprint of the Taylor & Francis Group, an informa business

© 2021 Hilary Moss

The right of Hilary Moss to be identified as author of this work has been asserted by her in accordance with sections 77 and 78 of the Copyright, Designs and Patents Act 1988.

British Library Cataloguing-in-Publication Data
A catalogue record for this book is available from the British Library

Library of Congress Cataloging-in-Publication Data
A catalog record has been requested for this book

ISBN: 978-0-367-34614-0 (hbk)
ISBN: 978-0-367-76534-7 (pbk)
ISBN: 978-0-429-32687-5 (ebk)

Typeset in Baskerville
by Newgen Publishing UK

Access the companion website: www.routledgemusicresearch.co.uk

For Martin, Luke and Eve Fahy and for the brave contributors to this book who live with serious health conditions.

Contents

List of figures

List of online files

Introduction

Chapter 1

Chapter 2

Chapter 3

Chapter 4

Chapter 5

Note:

The audio examples marked with ***** can be accessed via the online Routledge Music Research Portal: www.routledgemusicresearch.co.uk. Please enter the activation word **RRMusic** and your email address when prompted. You will immediately be sent an automated email containing an access token and instructions, which will allow you to log in to the site.

For the rest of the examples please refer to the links inside the book. Please note that websites can change beyond our control.

Foreword

While many of the elements of hospital care have changed and improved enormously over the millennia, an aspect lost since the sanctuary hospitals of the time of Hippocrates in ancient Greek culture is the importance of aesthetic supports, such as music, poetry and theatre, in healing. Modern hospitals are more often than not sterile and impersonal environments, delivering on the huge technical advances of modern medical science but neglecting the fuller picture of what it is to be human, ill and vulnerable. In so doing, they also miss out on drawing on the resilience of the human spirit which is often augmented and enhanced by personal and shared experiences of music and the arts.

Happily, there a growing movement to enhance hospital life for patients, visitors and staff with music and the arts: allied to this is an increasing research base showing why this is important, evidence of positive impacts, and insight into the elements that contribute to a person-centred approach to providing and replenishing aesthetic supports when attending hospital. Hilary Moss has been a pioneering leader in both providing musical enrichment in hospital settings and also in undertaking the research into what are the elements of aesthetic enrichment and how to characterise and develop the sophisticated art of arts curation in hospital settings.

Her background as a musician, music therapist, arts and health practitioner and researcher embedded in research and education contribute to a unique alliance of practical and innovative music programming with a critical eye on research and scholarship. This combination of factors means that this book is likely to be required reading for arts and health practitioners and directors, musicians, music therapists, and hospital-based clinicians and managers who are interested in broader approaches to quality of care and healing.

Martin Luther wrote that his heart was often solaced and refreshed by music when sick and weary. If that solace can happen in our private lives,

I welcome the insights and supports that Dr Moss provides in this book to ensure that such solace can also be found during our challenging journeys through the many spaces and elements of modern hospital care.

Prof Desmond O'Neill MD FRCPI
Trinity College Dublin

Acknowledgements

Many people inspired and informed this book.

The staff and service users at Tallaght University Hospital, especially Alison Baker-Kerrigan, Lucia Barnes and Clara Monahan from the National Centre for Arts and Health; the clinical teams at the Age Related Health Care Unit and the Renal Dialysis Unit and the hospital choir.

Music Therapists who taught me, shaped my practice, mentored and inspired me, including and especially Ann Sloboda, Gary Ansdell, Joanne Loewy, Amy Clement Cortez, Michael Silverman, Tessa Watson, Rachel Darnley-Smith, Alison Mahraj, Anna Maratos, Martin Fahy, Rebecca O'Connor, Bill Ahessy, Philippa Derrington, Claire Flower, Paula Higgins, Jessica O'Donoghue, Shane Cassidy, Wendy Magee, Sarah Hoskyns, Triona McCaffrey, Dee Gray, Karen Diamond and Katie Fitzpatrick.

My colleagues and friends at the Irish World Academy of Music and Dance, University of Limerick. Special mention to Dr Aileen Dillane, Prof Helen Phelan, Dr Kathleen Turner, Dr Mats Melin, Dr Sandra Joyce, Dr Diane Daly and Ms Pattie Punch who specifically encouraged and inspired sections of this book.

The graduates of the MA Music Therapy 2016–20, who provided insights and examples for this book, responded to drafts and taught me every day, including Siân Brown, Ryan Bolger, Paul Noonan, Daniel Dineen, Patrick Dalton, Elizabeth Helitzer, Fabian Joyce and Sabina Marr whose work and ideas appear in these pages. Also to brave undergraduate student Carol Freely who shared her story with me.

Art therapists Aimee O'Neill and Catherina Brady with whom I collaborated for many years.

Experts who gave their time and ideas freely and generously, including Prof Stephen Clift who generously read a whole draft, Dr Niamh Bohane, Dr Ian Wilson, Ailish Claffey, Dr Clare Donnellan, Dr Giorgos Tsiris, Prof Yuriko Saito, Prof Paul Crawford, Prof Brendan Kelly, Prof Shaun

O'Keeffe, Prof Bryan Lawson, Prof Dominic Harmon, Prof Tia DeNora, Fr John Kelly, Prof Dominic Harmon and Mr Jonathan Browner.

Musicians and performers who shared their time and expertise with service users and inspired me, including: Jane Bentley, Sophie Lee, Mairead O'Donnell, Kenneth Rice, Joachim Roewler, Malachy Robinson, Cathal Roche, Deirdre Moynihan, Ingrid Craigie, Sharon Murphy and the Irish Chamber Orchestra.

Above all I thank the service users who contributed to this book, especially Pacelli, Anne, Peter, Jo, Adrian and John and the service users in the Age Related Health Care Unit, TUH. There are too many of you to mention by name, but each one of you will never be forgotten. A special mention to Lynn Barrett, my youngest contributor, and her mum, for sharing her song with us. I wish you all health and well-being in the years to come.

Finally, especial thanks to Martin Fahy (who edited multiple drafts), Luke Fahy (especially for informing the section on music and torture) and Eve Fahy (who encouraged me constantly). Also Margaret and Tony Moss, Frances Holt and Ivan Moss for your constant encouragement and love.

Introduction

For the past twenty-five years my working life has been concerned, one way or another, with the relationship between the arts, health and well-being. On many occasions, I have seen how artistic engagement can result in measurable clinical gains, such as improvement in exercise levels, motivation, pain reduction or return to work. More often, though, my experience has underlined how the arts help in a less dramatic, and qualitatively different, way, not necessarily so helpfully measured as a healthcare 'intervention'.

As a musician, music therapist and arts manager, I have seen how the arts can offer moments of companionship, self-expression, hope and beauty. I have seen the arts kindle inspiration and insight and help others to perceive the ways that people retain, and gain power, in the face of debilitating illness. I have seen how the arts promote and sustain connection between people with illness and care staff, families and friends.

In what follows, I will tap into my 25 years of experience to focus on the role of music in healthcare settings, to showcase the value of music in situations of serious illness and extreme pain. Within this story are certain recurring themes that, I hope to demonstrate, are vital to all hospital-based music and health programmes. These themes are: the importance of recognising individuality and person-centred approaches; narrative, self-expression and meaning-making when coping with ill health; the connection between moments of music, beauty and hope; the importance of 'life-long' aesthetic experience (and with it the importance of 'aestheticised' care environments); the role of music as a means of communication when words are not available; the role of music as a simple, but significant, distraction from the pain and distress of illness; the deprivation and neglect caused by the absence of normal access to the arts and, finally, the challenges and institutional impediments to music within clinical care.

I also aim to challenge some of the assumptions made by music and health professionals – namely that music is always 'good for you', that it is never contraindicated and that any musical intervention is positive. I hope to provoke discussion by contending that health care spaces are normally places of aesthetic deprivation and neglect. Whilst much good work exists and must be recognised regarding design projects to humanise healthcare spaces, music can still be experienced as noise pollution and cause aesthetic injury (DeNora and Ansdell 2014). Engaging in music does not necessarily make you a happier or healthier person. I will also challenge music and health professionals to accept a variety of ways of working and rise above petty professional issues within the music and health field. Finally, I will argue that music must only be used in healthcare spaces by high quality professionals who are working with people for whom music engagement, in whatever form, is clinically indicated and welcomed by the person receiving care.

My aim will be, as much as possible, to feature the stories of specific people who, within clinical care settings and while contending with challenging illnesses, continue to engage creatively to live fully and meaningfully despite their health difficulties. In this way, this book is part of a recent trend in arts and health research and provision – one that highlights the importance of the person living with illness – and it understands music's role as a dynamic medium within clinical care ecologies.

The central questions that will be answered in this book are:

1. What can musical expression illuminate about service user experience in health care institutions?
2. Does music help people cope with serious illness and a hospital stay?
3. Can music improve the aesthetic environment of healthcare spaces or is music harmful?
4. To what extent, and in what circumstances, can music contribute to supporting clinical staff to provide high quality care?

The major arguments of this book are (1) The arts can help us understand the experiences of the person who is seriously ill, to improve care and help us cope with our caring roles. Music illuminates the experience of the person who is ill and can help care staff understand and support the person (2) Music helps people express themselves, cope and make meaning out of serious illness. Self-expression, creating community and cultivating hope are important aspects of coping with serious illness and music can contribute to these areas (3) Music contributes to creating a sense of choice and control in the healthcare environment, counteracting the negative aesthetics of institutional healthcare. Thus, music can contribute to quality of care and create an environment conducive to health and well-being. (4) Music can be damaging and unhelpful in healthcare. Working collaboratively and flexibly with clinical professionals is key to successful music-making in healthcare spaces.

John's story

This book starts with John's story. John was 78 years old when I met him. He was married with three adult daughters and had worked as an accountant until he retired. I met John in the last weeks of his life. He was receiving palliative care in hospital, following a major stroke. There were no more rehabilitative options for John. When I first met him, he was lying in bed with no ability to communicate verbally. He could only make groaning sounds. He needed 24-hour care, was PEG[1] fed, doubly incontinent and reportedly in pain. His wife Irene kept vigil by his bedside. She reported that he was a happy man, who enjoyed golf and quiet pursuits such as reading the newspaper and hill walking.

As part of my working life as a music therapist in an acute hospital, I always kept a few sessions free to 'pop in' to people in bed and offer some music. This was most often a receptive activity, whereby a service user would listen to me play music, and my visit aimed to create a moment of enjoyment, relaxation or solace. By offering music, I believed that I could offer a break or distraction from the bleak reality of ill health, institutional care and social isolation. A personally significant song or piece of music might transport a person, for a few minutes, to another mental space or time. The ability that music has to change the atmosphere of a room or evoke a memory is helpful in hospital. A piece of music can significantly transform the atmosphere of a ward, treatment room, clinic or hospital bedroom and can sometimes dissipate the tension between family members. It can offer a moment of beauty in a dark, difficult time of life and some people find music helps them transcend the everyday and grasp something spiritual. Some people I meet in hospital report that the music lifts their mood or is a brief distraction from pain, others find carefully chosen music relaxing, aiding interaction between fellow hospital residents and staff.

When I visited John, his wife Irene was in his room. She said yes, she would like to hear some music and thought John would too. John was unsettled and in pain and she thought maybe he would like to hear a song. I played a song he reportedly liked. Something in the moment after the song propelled me to offer Irene a song also. Perhaps I felt her grief, exhaustion and worry? I asked her if there was a song she would like to hear. She told me that as a couple, married for over forty years, they particularly loved Elvis Presley. As part of my professionalism as a music therapist, I made it my business to know one song (at least) by every major artist (without the need for sheet music or iPad) so that I could respond to requests spontaneously. The only song in my repertoire by Presley, however, was *Love me Tender*. I sang and played 'Love me tender' gently and quietly and Irene joined in. Irene stroked John's hand and his groaning quietened. Irene cried and said John had responded positively. The intimacy of this moment of singing and being together as a couple was an honour to witness.

Listen and watch online I.1: Elvis Presley, Love me tender www. youtube.com/watch?v=aoriFtRVGQs

This approach to engaging musically with people in hospital links closely to the body of work already documented regarding the role of music in everyday life (DeNora 2000). Firstly, music transformed the hospital bedroom for a few moments, just as music is used on an aeroplane to calm nervous passengers, or in aerobics classes to promote movement. Music is a powerful way to change the atmosphere of shops, restaurants, homes and workplaces (Jones and Schumacher 1992; McIntosh 2003). Secondly, music created a moment of emotional expression and intimacy. Irene cried and expressed her love for John. Thirdly, music calmed John and possibly reduced his experience of pain and discomfort. Music is often used in hospitals to calm people who may be agitated in a busy waiting room, or to create a tangible impression of competence where there is uncertainty during the process of treating a condition. A moment of music might offer a brief window of life and positivity in the dark experience of loss and trauma of illness. Choosing music to listen to offers a person in hospital a moment of choice and control in an environment in which decisions are often made without any input from the person receiving care.

Music is an important part of human life and culture and attracts a significant amount of private and public funding, attention and support. There is a strong body of evidence, particularly in the areas of acquired brain injury, pain management, adolescent mental health, care of older people and pre - surgery anxiety, that music can improve clinical outcomes. This book details relevant evidence bases where they exist and recent documents that have successfully summarised the evidence base regarding the contribution of the arts health and well-being. (Arts Council England 2018, 2020; Daykin 2020; Fancourt 2017; Fancourt and Finn 2019; All-Party Parliamentary Group on Arts, Health and Wellbeing 2017). While acknowledging the evidence that exists, and the role of the arts in positively impacting health and well-being, this book looks beyond the undeniable need for further quantitative evidence to ask a different set of questions.

In my experiences in hospital, engagement with music rarely dramatically changed clinical outcomes, physiological health status, requirements for pain medication, recovery time or costs of healthcare inputs. John's physical, psychological and cognitive health outcomes, for example, were not affected by my music therapy session and measuring his pain medication, length of hospital stay or other quantifiable measure would not have yielded useful 'proof' of the benefit of music therapy; and even if it did, it would be unlikely to persuade health service managers of the importance of music in palliative care. However, this access to music (and the arts) matters in healthcare settings because it contributes to humanising the environment, normalising the clinical and caring for the person. Engaging in individualised, personally important art-making contributes to improving care, quality of life, offering hope and motivation. These are the themes of this book.

This book aims to improve quality of care in hospitals and healthcare institutions. I hope to share the many ways that music can make a positive difference to the recovery and coping of people with serious illnesses in health care settings, as well as offering support to staff and family members. The emphasis of this work is to highlight the individuality of the person living with illness and to present how music quite literally brings humanity to the predominantly clinical, scientific arena of modern healthcare. However, this book also challenges popular notions that we need to 'prove the benefit' of music in hospital and professional hierarchies within music and health practice. Above all, I hope to demonstrate that music *does* matter, and give some inspiring examples and recommendations to make the most of music in healthcare settings.

Definitions and starting notes

In this book the term **service user** will be used to refer to any person who engages with health care professionals, settings and services. The terms 'patient', 'client' and 'service user' were all considered; all are far from ideal. Where possible, the person receiving healthcare is referred to as 'a person with…' but where a generic term is used 'service user' has been chosen.

This book focuses primary on **hospital**, as most of the experiences described arise from the contexts of acute and rehabilitation hospitals, as well as extended care for older people and mental health in-patient care. Whilst the term hospital is used frequently, the points made in this book are applicable to any building where health services are delivered, including community-based healthcare facilities, nursing homes, primary or tertiary care settings, in-patient, outpatient or day centre services.

The definition of **arts** used in this book is that of The Arts Council of Ireland. The Arts Act 2003 defines the arts as 'any creative or interpretative expression (whether traditional or contemporary) in whatever form, and includes, in particular, visual arts, theatre, literature, music, dance, opera, film, circus and architecture, and includes any medium when used for those purposes' (Government of Ireland 2003; The Arts Council 2006, 2010).

The term **aesthetics** is also used in this book. Terms such as 'arts', 'aesthetics' and 'culture' are contested words that are notoriously difficult to define (Davies 2005). The definition of aesthetics used is *An attempt to theorise about art, to explain what it is and why it matters* (Graham 1997). For the purpose of this book, therefore, aesthetics refers to the philosophy of arts and the role the arts play in society. It encompasses all art forms as well as broader issues such as the physical environment and everyday experiences related to beauty and art (Saito 2008).

Arguments continue about what constitutes 'art', for example whether popular and mass art are 'art', and some definitions of art can seem somewhat narrow and elitist (Davies 2005). Similarly, what constitutes music therapy, music and health and musical enrichment are all open to interpretation. This book wishes not to constrain the arts by reigning in and limiting them within narrow definitions or hierarchies. This book thus uses the term aesthetics, as per the definition above, as a broad reaching umbrella term to encompass all art forms and aesthetic experiences.

This book focuses on **music** as the art form within the author's expertise. However, occasionally other art forms are referred to where excellent examples demonstrate the issues being discussed. The author contends that many of the points made in this book are relatable to any arts/creative activity or intervention in healthcare spaces and can be applied to other arts engagement for health and well-being.

Music therapy is defined in this book as the clinical and evidence-based use of music interventions to accomplish individualised goals within a therapeutic relationship by a credentialed professional who has completed an approved music therapy programme (AMTA 2017).

A final definition is important for this book. **Arts in health** is a term with myriad definitions within the healthcare sector. For the purposes of this book, the term Arts in Health is used (as opposed to arts and health) in keeping with current research regarding terms and definitions (Sonke et al. 2017). However, the definition I offer here is from The Arts Council England, whereby 'Arts and Health' is defined as arts based activities that aim to improve individual and community health and healthcare delivery and which enhance the environment by providing artwork or performances (The Arts Council England 2007). The field of arts in healthcare that I inhabit embraces a wide range of practices including medical humanities, design aspects of healthcare, arts in hospice/end of life care, arts therapies and arts and aging (Brenner 2003).

Much has already been written about the role of music in healthcare settings, and this book stands on the shoulders of many giants of music and music therapy in healthcare spaces. This book is necessarily made of my own perspective and stories. The chapter titles represent key themes from my reflection of what matters most for service users – namely the importance of listening, telling my story, avoiding negative musical experiences and the positive benefits of music in hospital. Professional issues are addressed in the final chapter. In keeping with the marriage between music and health in this book, each chapter title is also linked to a musical term.

Above all, it is hoped that this book contributes to, and generates, discussion, reflection and awareness of how music can be used effectively to improve quality of care and support people living with serious illness, their clinicians and their families.

> I'm not sure I can tell the truth, I can only tell what I know.
>
> (Pollack, 2010)

Note

1 PEG stands for percutaneous endoscopic gastrostomy, a procedure in which a flexible feeding tube is placed through the abdominal wall and into the stomach. PEG allows nutrition, fluids and/or medications to be put directly into the stomach, bypassing the mouth and esophagus.

Further reading

The further reading offered in this introduction offers a variety of texts to set the current scene regarding music, health and well-being practice and research. Suggested reading can never be comprehensive. All reading lists are suggested as stepping off points for further exploration on the part of the reader.

All-Party Parliamentary Group on Arts, Health and Wellbeing (2017) *Creative health: the arts for health and wellbeing.* London. Retrieved from www.artshealthandwellbeing. org.uk/appg-inquiry/Publications/Creative_Health_Inquiry_Report_2017.pdf.

Ansdell, G. (2014) *How music helps in music therapy and everyday life.* Farnham: Ashgate.

Arts Council England (2018) *Arts and culture in health and well-being and in the criminal justice system: a summary of evidence.* London: Arts Council England Retrieved from www.artscouncil.org.uk/publication/arts-and-culture-health-and-wellbeing-and-criminal-justice-system-summary-evidence.

Arts Council England (2020) Arts, culture and wellbeing. Retrieved from www.artscouncil.org.uk/developing-creativity-and-culture/arts-culture-and-wellbeing.

Clift, S. and Camic, P. M.(2016) *Oxford textbook of creative arts, health, and wellbeing: international perspectives on practice, policy and research.* Oxford: Oxford University Press.

Daykin, N. (2020) *Arts, health and well-being: a critical perspective on research, policy and practice.* Abingdon: Routledge.

DeNora, T. (2000) *Music in everyday life.* Cambridge: Cambridge University Press.

DeNora T. and Ansdell G. (2014) What can't music do? *Psychology of Well-Being: Theory, Research and Practice* 4. doi:10.1186/s13612-014-0023-6.

Fancourt, D. (2017) *Arts in health designing and researching interventions*. Oxford: Oxford University Press.

Fancourt, D., and Finn, S. (2019) *What is the evidence on the role of the arts in improving health and well-being? A scoping review*. World Health Organisation, available: www. euro.who.int/en/publications/abstracts/what-is-the-evidence-on-the-role-of-the-arts-in-improving-health-and-well-being-a-scoping-review-2019.

MacDonald, R.A.R. (2013) Music, health, and well-being: a review. *International journal of qualitative studies on health and well-being*, 8, 20635. doi:10.3402/qhw. v8i0.2063.

Stickley, T., and Clift, S., eds. (2017) *Arts, health and wellbeing: a theoretical inquiry for practice*. Newcastle upon Tyne: Cambridge Scholars.

AMTA www.musictherapy.org/about/quotes/.

BAMT www.bamt.org.

References

The All-Party Parliamentary Group on Arts, Health and Wellbeing (2017) *Creative health: the arts for health and wellbeing*. London, available: www.artshealthand well-being.org.uk/appg-inquiry/Publications/Creative_Health_Inquiry_Report_2017.pdf.

AMTA (2017) What is music therapy?, available: www.musictherapy.org/about/quotes/.

The Arts Council (2006) *The public and the arts*. Dublin: The Arts Council.

The Arts Council (2010) *Arts and health policy*. Dublin: The Arts Council.

The Arts Council England (2007) *The arts, health and wellbeing*. Liverpool: John Moores University.

Arts Council England (2018) *Arts and culture in health and well-being and in the criminal justice system: a summary of evidence*. London: Arts Council England, available: www. artscouncil.org.uk/publication/arts-and-culture-health-and-wellbeing-and-criminal-justice-system-summary-evidence.

Arts Council England (2020) Arts, culture and wellbeing, available: www.artscouncil. org.uk/developing-creativity-and-culture/arts-culture-and-wellbeing.

American Music Therapy Association (2017) Definitions and quotes about music therapy, available: www.musictherapy.org/about/quotes.

Brenner, S. (2003) *Report on the arts in healthcare symposium*. National Endowment for the Arts, Washington DC, available: https://nasaa-arts.org/wp-content/uploads/2017/03/B-Health-SymposSumm.pdf.

Davies, S. (2005) Definitions of Art. In B. Gaut and D. McIver Lopes, eds., *The Routledge companion to aesthetics*, 2nd ed. Abingdon: Routledge, 227–41.

Daykin, N. (2020) *Arts, health and well-being: a critical perspective on research, policy and practice*. Abingdon: Routledge.

DeNora, T. (2000) *Music in everyday life*. Cambridge: Cambridge University Press.

DeNora T, and Ansdell G. (2014) What can't music do? *Psychology of Well-Being: Theory, Research and Practice* 4. doi:10.1186/s13612-014-0023-6.

Fancourt, D. (2017) *Arts in health designing and researching interventions*. Oxford: Oxford University Press.

Fancourt, D., and Finn, S. (2019) *What is the evidence on the role of the arts in improving health and well-being? A scoping review* World Health Organisation, available: www. euro.who.int/en/publications/abstracts/what-is-the-evidence-on-the-role-of-the-arts-in-improving-health-and-well-being-a-scoping-review-2019.

Government of Ireland (2003) *The arts act.* Ireland: Government of Ireland, available: www.irishstatutebook.ie/eli/2003/act/24/enacted/en/html.

Graham, G. (1997) *Philosophy of the arts, an introduction to aesthetics.* London: Routledge.

Jones, S.C., and Schumacher, T.G. (1992) Muzak: On functional music and power. *Critical Studies in Mass Communication*, 9(2), 156–69. doi:10.1080/15295039209366822.

McIntosh, I.B. (2003) Flying-related stress. In R. Bor, ed., *Passenger behaviour.* Abingdon: Routledge 17–31.

Pollack, E. (2010) *Creative nonfiction: a guide to form, content, and style, with readings.* Boston: Wadsworth Cengage Learning.

Saito, Y. (2008) *Everyday aesthetics.* Oxford: Oxford University Press.

Sonke, J., Lee, J., Rollins, J., Carytsas, R., Imus, S., Lambert, P., … Spooner, H. (2017) *White paper: talking about arts in health.* Retrieved from Gainsville, Florida: https://arts.ufl.edu/academics/center-for-arts-in-medicine/resources/talking-about-arts-in-health/executive-summary/.

1   Listening

When I began working as a hospital musician, I felt like a fish out of water. The world of performing, creating, rehearsing and practising every nuance of a piece of music was replaced with a different sound world – beeps, machines, loud speaker announcements, the sound of staff walking fast up and down the ward, conversations at the nurses station, laughter, serious discussions, the sound of wheels – wheelchairs, trolley beds, supplies being transferred, linen and bins carts and hospital food trolleys. The sounds of tears, pain, grieving. The sounds of televisions that no-one was listening to, family visits, the busy atrium where 2,000 staff and 4,000 service users passed through every morning. Occasionally the sound of loud voices complaining, arguments between family members, abuse shouted at reception staff. The sound of emergency sirens as the ambulance approached emergency rooms, the helicopter occasionally landing on the H-pad, the grass being mown, the electronic numbering system calling the next service user into phlebotomy or the outpatient clinic, the sound of MRI scanners, x-ray machines, staff discussions in corridors or fast, efficient footsteps.

The sound world of hospital is often chaotic, noisy and disjointed. The sound world of the 15-piece swing band, in which I played trombone, is ordered and systematic. Everything fits together, resolves together, the peaks and troughs are journeyed through together. The Glen Miller band in online clip 1 exemplifies the ordered, systematic and highly sophisticated sound of 15 musicians playing together. The musicians are listening, anticipating the other players moves and perfectly synchronising their breathing, physical, cognitive and emotional reactions in order to play together in the same style, appropriate dynamic range and intensity.

> Listen and watch online 1.1: Glenn Miller Orchestra, In the Mood
> www.youtube.com/watch?v=UgkadSCPtbU

This chapter will explore the need for careful listening by artists and health providers to fully assess and provide what service users want and need. This may involve curbing a tendency to programme music programmes without fully consulting service users. The chapter contends that musicians are expert listeners and can offer reflection on clinical listening. The predominance of participative music-making (to the exclusion of simply listening to music) is also noted with a brief review of some of the benefits of music listening for health and well-being.

As a hospital music therapist, I regularly attended ward rounds, team meetings and clinical case review meetings. Sometimes the multi-disciplinary team felt as connected as the Glen Miller band, at other times the team was disjointed and unconnected, rarely meeting, communicating or listening. Even functional healthcare teams can find it a challenge to find time for genuine communication or reflection. In my experience, healthcare teams can often be disjointed, communication can be poor and overall performance suffers. My role as a music therapist was often viewed as adjunct to the core team, and my involvement in the team thus would feel disjointed. A visiting music therapist, offering a group programme for clients in a nursing home, for example, can feel very disconnected from the team. The power balance between professionals was often overt, and 'lower' staff deferred to the opinion of the chiefs of the team. A music ensemble also has a hierarchy but even those with very few notes to play commit to their contribution, and this is understood as crucial to the whole rather than dispensable or of secondary importance to another.

Before my hospital life, I spent my time training to be a musician. This time included listening to Beethoven symphonies and playing long low notes to warm up on my trombone for 20 minutes before performance or practice. Once I started work in a hospital, such quiet attention to detail was replaced with highly efficient meetings, typically 5–10 minutes of key information exchange between busy clinical staff. The intense concentration required at an orchestral rehearsal was replaced by the intense focus given to a family meeting, a clinical review meeting or a planning meeting for a new design section of the building. The language of the arts that I was steeped in, such as describing, reflecting, illuminating, quoting, was replaced with scientific lab tests, statistical results and formulae that I did not understand.

Working as a clinical music therapist was a journey from the arts to science and back again. For those who work at the intersection between arts and health, there is a new language to be learned, a cultural shift that takes place. Without this mutual understanding, creative, original and helpful arts projects in healthcare environments cannot happen. In my experience, science and the humanities do not exist in an 'either/or' situation and the split between these worlds in current society is artificial and unhelpful (Roche et al. 2018). Engel's biopsychosocial model of medicine went a long way towards repairing the artificial split between aspects of our health, but the role of the arts in healthcare remains considered as a dispensable luxury, the icing on the cake, inessential but nice if you have time or energy to bother with adding it to the healthcare environment (Engel 1977; Edgar and Pattison 2006).

What has become apparent to me, as a musician, music therapist and manager of arts and health programmes in a large city hospital, is that the most important thing is listening.

Failure to listen in healthcare settings

Listening is a buzz word in health service delivery. In 2013 one of the biggest failures in UK NHS care was revealed. Between 400 and 1,200 service users died as a result of poor care over the 50 months between January 2005 and March 2009 at Stafford hospital, a small district general hospital in Staffordshire (Campbell 2013). A report published on 6 February 2013 (the fifth report into the scandal) revealed the horrifying evidence, and 'Mid Staffs' became a byword for a lack of NHS care at its most negligent (Francis 2013). It is often described as the worst hospital care scandal of recent times. In 2013 Sir Ian Kennedy, the chairman of the Healthcare Commission and the regulator of NHS care standards at the time, said it was the most shocking scandal he had investigated (Lancet 2014).

The failure of care in the Mid Staffordshire scandal was arguably a failure of listening. Robert Francis QC, author of the 2013 report, stated that: '(the Trust Board) did not listen sufficiently to its patients and staff… in part the consequence of allowing a focus on reaching national access targets, achieving financial balance at the cost of delivering acceptable standards of care' (Francis 2013). Criticism was made of the institutional management and culture, which ascribed more weight to positive information than information raising cause for concern, punished whistleblowers and failed to act when informed of issues that required action.

In recent years, the NHS has regularly stipulated the need for listening to be a core element of good healthcare and this is reflected in many national health policies in this century. A 2013 white paper by NHS Wales, for example, stipulates the need for listening to become 'a planned activity' and several national policy documents have focused in recent years on listening and positive communication in order to reduce complaints and improve service user experience of health care delivery (Williams 2013).

Musicians are expert listeners

As a musician, I am steeped in the art of listening. From a young age, musicians practise for hours, listening intently to learn to play better. They take apart large sections of music to rework miniscule phrases, even individual notes. The musician returns to problematic sections and hones in on significant moments. They switch from detailed listening to listening to the overall direction of the music. When a musician plays with others in an ensemble, they listen intently to several lines of music at once and attend to the music of others.

Orchestral musicians listen to optimise delivery of their part of the music. By listening they can shape their own contribution to match perfectly and complement the other sounds – the dynamics, the timing, the shape of the phrase for example. They also listen to ensure that the sound of their instrument contributes to the music as a whole. Figure 1.1 shows a typical trombone part for an orchestral player. As a trombonist, I often spend large amounts of rehearsal time counting bars of rest! Nonetheless, this acute listening to long sections before the loud, dramatic entry of the brass, is crucial in making my small part count.

If a health service team are not listening to each other, how can they make their contribution fit in the overall whole? If they are not listening to the service user and their family, how can they meet their needs effectively? And if a music therapist or other adjunct therapist is not integrated as part of the clinical team, attending discussions, family meetings and case reviews, how can their contribution be relevant and helpful to the overall case? Performance and optimum care must surely suffer. Is it possible that a music therapist in the clinical team can offer something particularly useful with regards to listening?

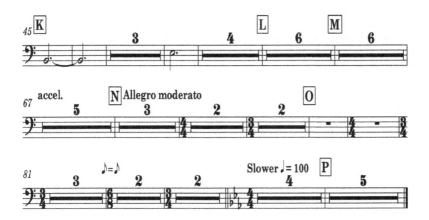

Figure 1.1 Typical trombone part in an orchestra

Mowat and colleagues contend that there are three types of listening in healthcare organisations: (1) listening to obtain information to optimize service delivery; (2) listening to obtain information that helps understand the relationship between the person and the organization and (3) listening for its own sake without an external objective. In the third type of listening, there is no purpose for listening, the listener is not trying to achieve something, but rather allowing the person to tell their story for their own well-being (Mowat et al. 2013). However, listening is complex. Professional skills such as accurate listening are neither visible nor easy to measure. Clinicians are taught to listen rigorously as part of their education and training, for example the 'golden minute' in consultations where doctors are encouraged to allow a service user at least a minute to say what they want (Beckman and Frankel 1984; Awdish and Berry 2017; Coope 2020). Listening is a position, a stance, an attitude, a choice, not a passive act (Stickley and Freshwater 2006). It is a craft that can be developed through supervised practice. Service users tend to be more dissatisfied with poor communication than any other part of their care, a fact which warrants attention during clinical training (Mallett and Dougherty 2000; Keatings et al. 2002).

Music therapists have time to listen

One of the luxuries of working as a music therapist in a hospital setting is time. I have time to spend an hour with my client, listening, offering opportunities for self-expression, validation of identity and offering support. It is a privileged position in a busy health service environment. Stickley and Freshwater observe that in the rush of modern health care practice, there is arguably little encouragement or time for self-reflection in nursing (Stickley and Freshwater 2006). Music, however, affords a unique opportunity for listening. The very crux of music therapy is to say to the client, through music, 'I am listening to you'. The music we play can validate the individuality of the person who chooses it, but even in non-verbal musical exchanges music therapists can acknowledge the communication by attuning to the music the person offers. We use three specific musical techniques to achieve this: mirroring, matching and dialoguing. In each of these the emphasis is on attuning to the client's music, creating a musical exchange and reflecting back to the client what they are communicating through the music.

As a teacher of student music therapists, I emphasise the importance of active listening. A common mistake in music therapy is to start to play music for a client before the client has a chance to express themselves or make a choice. For example, we might offer a client a choice of instruments and they might choose to play a drum. Even if the therapist waits for the client to play first, they routinely jump in too quickly and start to play with them. Better to wait and listen and only join in when you have something useful to say. If two people improvising is a non-verbal conversation, then the therapist is taking over in this instance, being supportive but over eager. The client is saying on their drum 'I want to say something' but the therapist is leaping in, saying 'Great, yes, let's talk. What do you want to say? Is it this? Or that? Can I help?'. We often overwhelm the unique expression of the client whose voice is drowned out by the music therapist's eagerness to perform!

Time and again I have found it more beneficial to wait, listen and pause before responding. One of two things can happen. First, the client will say more about themselves. They might change instrument, intensity or pace. They may surprise the therapist. They are free to bring their own voice on the drum into the room. The second possibility is that they will not say more, but the therapist, by listening says 'I am listening and when I play I will try to support you to say more, but I will be careful not to drown you out'.

The following two online examples demonstrate music therapists Rebecca O'Connor and Bill Ahessy improvising with clients who find verbal communication extremely difficult. Both examples are highly sophisticated music conversations, in which the therapist demonstrates attuning to the client, matching intensity, dynamics, pace, tonality, timbre and rhythm and musical dialogue.

Listen and watch online 1.2: Ben with Rebecca O'Connor* for all audio files marked with * in this chapter, see List of online files for access details on p. ix.

This extract is from a young boy's music therapy session whilst he was at the National Rehabilitation Hospital following an acquired brain injury. Music therapy was an integral aspect of his interdisciplinary rehabilitation programme. As a result of his injury he was nonverbal, and had physical limitations, cognitive difficulties and behavioural issues. In other situations he was displaying frustration at not understanding what was happening to him and at losing control of so much in his life. In this extract he displays an awareness that he is in control of both the therapist's music and the interaction and is working towards avoiding the ending of the session by trying hard to have the 'last word' with his music. In this session he has also just realised that he is able to convey his emotions through vocal sounds and the musical instruments and appears delighted at being able to express himself and take part in musical conversations. It is a wonderful example of the therapist attuning to the musical communication of the client.

Listen and watch online 1.3: Mary with Bill Ahessy*

Initially Mary (the client) found it difficult to engage in improvisation due to attention deficit and verbal perseveration. As the therapy sessions developed she began to listen and focus more, exploring creatively and again this is an example of client and therapist attuning through active listening and music making. For more information see Ahessy, 2017.

Active listening and the musician's perspective

Gerard Egan developed the S.O.L.E.R. system of active listening as a way to physically demonstrate the therapist's interest and engagement (Egan 2018). His model is used today in clinical counselling and professional settings worldwide and is useful in any situation as a baseline for better listening. Observational studies indicate that when active listening principles are used, people feel more understood and satisfied with the communication (Weger et al. 2014). Egan's theory depicts the most effective body language to employ to make others feel cared for. SOLER is an acronym that stands for:

- S (Square): Face squarely; by doing this it shows you are involved.
- O (Open): Keep an open posture: this means not crossing arms and legs. It makes people feel engaged and welcome.
- L (Lean): By leaning forward when a person is talking to you, it shows you are involved and listening to what they have to say.
- E (Eye Contact): Use good eye contact. Your gaze shows that you're listening and not distracted.
- R (Relax): It's important to stay calm and avoid fidgeting when a person is talking to show you are focused.

In the busyness of modern life, much of our time is taken up with passive listening. There is so much background noise in our lives (literal and figurative) that it becomes difficult to maintain active listening. Healthcare environments are pressurised workplaces. A consultant rheumatologist I worked with described his outpatient clinic as follows:

> I have 60 service users on a list to see this afternoon from 2pm. I'm lucky if I finish by 6 or 7pm without a break. I want to listen and support these people, but all I have time for is to hear about their physical issues and review their medication. This is far from satisfactory and I rely on other clinicians to pick up the pieces if someone is upset in my

clinic. If I let the emotion get to me, I would not be standing after 60 consultations, the stress for everyone can be overwhelming.

The world-renowned violinist Joshua Bell famously went unnoticed when he busked in a metro station, making only $32 in a day. People were so busy they failed to really hear the violinist in the station (Service 2007). We are so overloaded with sounds, as well as concerns for future events, that listening is difficult. Passive listening makes it difficult for the real 'music' to break through and make an impact. In therapeutic situations we may find ourselves reloading rather than listening, that is, we are preparing to speak in response while the person talks, rather than really listening to what they say.

> Many who write about active listening say it is the same skill with pieces of music and with people; you are developing a relationship through repeated active listening and the process of getting to know both music and people are remarkably similar. Active listening is specifically making listening the primary activity and doing nothing else. Just listen.
> (Huff 2016)

Huff (2016) recommends the following approach to active listening (whether listening to music or people):

- Start small: 3 mins active music listening as opposed to actively listening to a Wagner opera of 17 hours
- Focus on specific elements: Listen to the bass line of Paul McCartney's Nowhere Man. Active listening to this one line, repeatedly, will allow you to hear how amazing that piece of music is. 'That's what active listening does – it leads to intimacy, understanding, and appreciation' (Huff 2016)
- Repetition: Listen over and over. Listen to what's familiar but then listen again to what's unfamiliar.
- Take notes after: Active listening requires full attention.
- Open yourself stylistically: All of the great musical artists have been exceptional active listeners. One thing that many of them have in common is their willingness to branch out and draw inspiration from other genres and styles of music different than their own. Be willing as a clinician to extend your creativity, to open yourself to new experiences and approaches.

Listening to a new piece of music involves welcoming something different and new. How we view this depends on elements of the music itself but also our cultural norms, our expectations and our prior acquired knowledge of music (Warren 2014). The listener's context greatly affects whether a sound is received and perceived to be music or noise pollution (Scruton 2009). A music therapist, Martin, describes actively listening to clients with dementia. Some staff, he reports, describe the conversation as meaningless, a jumble of cognitive confusion and memory loss. But he hears the person with dementia as if they are reading a poem. He believes there is a poetry in the 'ramblings' of an incoherent person (and of course poetry has musical characteristics). There is often an atmosphere, an emotional communication, even if the words don't immediately make sense. For example, he observes that for one client, her verbal wanderings on the weather forecast could be understood as a metaphor for control. Perhaps we sometimes, as clinicians, fall foul of listening to the music of the person's story in the clinic, and instead hear the noise, busyness, stress and rush around us as we try to pick out key facts?

Clinical listening – what can music offer?

Numerous studies have been undertaken to explore the role of creativity and arts as learning activities with trainee doctors. Whilst the evidence base is limited, qualitative findings indicate that participants find arts-based approaches effective in learning listening and visual attention skills. In a study of neurology students, for example, trainees noticed they were better at recognising multiple points of view in encounters with service users following a course of visual art observation and narrative medicine classes. Prior to the session, 63 per cent of participants rated their listening skills as above average while 45 per cent rated their observation skills as above average. After the session, 80 per cent of participants rated their listening and observation skills as above average. Comments on the course cited the importance of reflection, focused attention, awareness of multiple perspectives, and appreciation of colleagues (Harrison and Chiota-McCollum 2019).

Ho and Srivatava (2019) argue that interwoven into the art of medicine sits communication skills – how a physician listens to the person, builds space for their concerns to be heard and dialogues about solutions. Evidence-based medicine and the most up-to-date medications may be able to help physical manifestations of pain, but the art of listening should not be underestimated in its ability to help a person heal. 'Sometimes, and especially in cases when medications cannot help, the art of listening is the only tool we have to offer' (Ho and Srivastava 2019).

A study using jazz improvisation as a training tool for medical doctors explained that the programme aimed to expose students to situations that were nonlinear and emergent, requiring listening, inductive thinking, and complex adaptive decision-making (Haidet et al. 2017). These were seen as

common characteristics of medicine and jazz. Medical students in this programme studied jazz music, with a focus on four communication skills: balancing communicative structure with communicative freedom when talking
with patients; listening for deep meanings in patients' communications;
developing one's own authentic 'voice' as a communicator; and effectively
using space (including communicative, physical, psychological, and top-
ical) in the medical encounter. For example, students listened to jazz singers
performing the same song and discussed the use of one's own voice to communicate authentically. Much of the medical literature suggests that students
are acculturated into a hierarchical environment wherein 'command and
control' decision-making is the norm, and many adopt the belief that medicine is characterised by linear, cause-and-effect problems best solved only by
algorithmic and deductive thinking (Haidet et al. 2017).

This is, I believe, the nub of what doctors and musicians have in common.
Despite attempts to regulate and be absolute, medicine is full of messy
grey areas. Music therapists often work in these grey areas, for example
with people receiving palliative care who need more than pharmaco-
logical treatment, for those living with long-term chronic conditions such as
chronic pain, arthritis, mental health issues, who need complex programmes
of supports in order to rehabilitate and recover to their optimum level.
Musicians live in a subjective, interpretative space where there is always
room for creative interpretation about how to express and play the notes.

Imhof and Janusik (2006) categorise listening into four types: a relationship building activity, to organise information, to learn and integrate
information or a critical endeavour. Individual proficiency can vary and
identifying our own listening style may be very useful, especially our ability
to undertake therapeutic listening and appreciative listening (Imhof and
Janusik 2006). Stickley argues that before we can successfully listen to others
we must learn the art of listening to self (Stickley and Freshwater 2006).
Self-care involves listening to ourselves, and clinicians need to prioritise time
for their own health and well-being.

My starting point for this book is that we often begin in the wrong place.
Listening is the key attribute that we need in bringing musical and creative
endeavours into healthcare spaces, and arguably a heightened awareness of
listening in all clinical professionals will improve clinical delivery, management and quality of care in the healthcare organisation.

Celia's story

Celia had a stroke and was resident in a medical ward for older people in
a busy London acute hospital. She was a single woman, age 68, who had
worked as an administrator in local factory. I worked as music therapist and

researcher on her ward. Most service users were unable to move independently, and many had complex medical needs and limited verbal responses.

The ward was the worst ward I ever worked on. I spent two days on the ward, observing and *listening*, watching how service users were treated and experiencing life alongside them. Staff seemed positively unkind to visitors, disinterested in visiting staff like me and attended to the basics of care only. The TV, I remember, was on all day, blaring out whatever was the channel of choice at the start of the day, without reference to whether anyone was listening. One day I visited, and children's TV was playing, the TV left unattended and neglected until it showed wholly inappropriate programmes.

Celia was referred to music therapy as she was isolating herself on the ward and seemed low in mood. I invited Celia to accompany me to the music therapy room. She said she loved music and came willingly. However, when she entered the room and saw the piano, drums and several percussion instruments she immediately stopped and said she didn't play any instruments and didn't want to. She didn't want to sing either. During the first session – always an assessment session with any new client – I tried various ideas to engage her musically, but all my usual attempts were met with a gentle resistance. Celia did not want to engage in music-making or singing. We talked about the repertoire she enjoyed instead. The first session was purely this: conversation about music she enjoyed. I sang 'You'll never walk alone' as she was a Liverpool FC supporter. In the second session I began to wonder what I could offer Celia. She came willingly to the room and talked further about loving to listen to symphonies, especially Beethoven's Third. We agreed, on my suggestion, that I would bring a CD of this work to the next session.

What followed were twelve sessions where each week we listened to a major symphony. I brought a CD player and the relevant CD. Celia and I listened together and talked a little at the beginning and the end of the session. Three important things happened – firstly, Celia told me she loved the quiet space of the music therapy room. She found the ward noisy, difficult to manage and quite stressful. She loved the space and privacy of this room. I realised that this was enough of a therapeutic aim, to enable Celia to have a quiet space on the ward for an hour each week. From then on, one of my missions in all healthcare spaces I worked in, was to find or create quiet spaces and to keep these on the agenda for service users whenever involved in planning new healthcare services. Secondly, Celia told me that she had a huge CD collection at home. Celia was moving to a nursing home from hospital as she was no longer able to take care of herself and had few family members willing to assist her. However, she seemed totally disengaged with the process, and when I asked her if she would bring her extensive music collection with her, she was disinterested and non-committal. She had made no attempt to bring in music from home to listen to in hospital either. When I suggested a friend might bring in some of her CDs to hospital, she was similarly unwilling or unable to think about whether this might be possible. This short piece of important work with Celia made me realise that hospital or nursing home could be so much better if one had their personally important objects, activities and passions around them. Celia's quality of life would have improved tremendously with a quiet space on the ward and her CD collection (or any collection) available to her. This experience made me wonder why, in hospital, there is such a neglect of the aesthetic, cultural and leisure pursuits that make life meaningful for people? (Moss and O'Neill 2014; Moss et al. 2015). Finally, Celia made me realise the importance of listening. Listening to music for its own sake, listening to the person receiving care rather than trying to 'fix' them or offer a solution that we think is helpful. Listening to what matters to the person and setting goals that they want to reach is very important.

Listening to music for health and well-being

Music listening can be an effective intervention for service users in medical settings to improve physical measures including heart rate, respiratory rate, anxiety and pain (Bradt et al. 2013a; Bradt et al. 2013b; Bradt et al. 2016; Silverman et al. 2016; Selle and Silverman 2020). Since many people in hospital feel unwell and tired, with low physical capability or motivation and raised levels of stress and anxiety, a receptive (i.e. listening) music experience may be desirable (Miller and O'Callaghan 2010). Active co-creation of music requires energy and risk taking capabilities (Silverman et al. 2016) whereas listening may provide entertainment, diversion, intense emotional experiences, cognitive and physical stimulation and discharge of negative feelings without active participation (Saarikallio 2012; Silverman 2019). Listening to music has received relatively sparse attention in the literature, with more studies focusing on active participation in creative arts (Moss et al. 2012). Spintge (2004) coined the phrase *Music Medicine* to refer to clinicians prescribing listening to music for relaxation and distraction from pain (Spintge 2004; Zengin et al. 2013). Music listening is a common behaviour that people can use to maintain an internal state, manage negative emotions, enhance positive emotions and improve emotion states (Sakka and Juslin 2018; Silverman 2019).

Studies emphasise the importance of service user personal preference and choice of music. Evidence exists that this makes for a more effective music listening intervention (Huang et al. 2010; Chang et al. 2011; Hanser 2014). Music preference is key to music therapy practice (and is often not a feature of other music listening approaches) and Standley's meta-analysis further demonstrates that when music therapists utilise the service user's preferred music, the effect sizes of benefits such as pain or anxiety reduction are higher (Standley 2000). Preferred or self-chosen music is likely to be especially proficient at reducing pain as self-chosen music is already liked, which provides an easily achievable sustained attention and entrainment (Mitchell and MacDonald 2006; Mitchell et al. 2008; Garza-Villarreal et al. 2014; Fidler and Mikzsa 2020).

The analgesic effect of listening to music may be secondary to cognitive and emotional effects that arise from listening to music, namely distraction from the pain, pleasantness, and pleasure, memory evoked emotions and relaxation (Garza-Villarreal et al. 2017). Selle and Silverman (2017) conducted a randomised feasibility study investigating the effects of a single session of music therapy using listening to personally preferred music for cardiovascular patients. They studied mood and pain. The researchers found that this approach can have immediate positive effects on anxiety, depression and pain. However, they concluded that little is known as to how service users perceive and experience this music and why receptive music listening may be an effective intervention (Selle and Silverman 2017, 2020).

Listening to music while working in hospital

A 2020 systematic review of studies on music in operating theatres concluded that beneficial effects of music on surgical performance have been observed and outweigh the negative effects, but noise distraction is also observed in some studies (Ullmann et al. 2008; Makama et al. 2010; El Boghdady and Ewalds-Kvist 2020). Self-chosen music is of course preferable in theatre as surgeons and their teams need to like the music they use as background support. A study of nurses indicated that soothing music was an effective stress reduction technique (Lai and Li 2011). Research in this area is relatively limited and there is potential to increase the usefulness of music in reducing health care workers' stress. A recent body of work focuses on the benefit of workplace choirs for health service staff (Vaag et al. 2013; Moss and O'Donoghue 2019).

How musical listening helps – Gerry's story

Gerry is a 31-year-old man who experienced a catastrophic hypoxic brain injury caused by a reduced supply of oxygen to his brain following a cardiac arrest. Gerry has no volitional movement, is visually impaired and has a severe cognitive deficit. He was admitted to hospital three years post-diagnosis as he was displaying severe distress, crying for long periods of time and shouting. Gerry would become distressed when approached or touched making it very difficult for staff to care for him in the long-term care facility. This story involves the work of music therapist Rebecca O'Connor at the National Rehabilitation Hospital, Dublin and is an example of excellent care through skilled musical listening.

Gerry underwent an extensive musical assessment called MATADOC (Magee and O'Kelly 2015) as part of his overall assessment process to contribute towards his diagnosis but also to identify any significant responses to musical stimulation. The music therapists presented a variety of sounds, including several different musical instruments and personally meaningful songs. Music was used in a sensitive, controlled manner as per the MATADOC protocol. The assessment process detailed the specific sounds and music Gerry was most responsive to by analysing video recordings and monitoring consistent, reproducible responses to the auditory stimuli.

It was identified that Gerry appeared to calm and his crying gradually reduced during clinical improvisation when the music therapist played the flute, matching the music to the rate of his breathing patterns and body movements, in the key of D minor – reflecting the pitch, sounds and intensity of his vocalisations. The music therapist produced music aiming to reflect any observed changes in Gerry's behaviour, the emotional quality of his sounds and his movements. Initially up to 20 minutes of playing the flute in this specific way was required before Gerry displayed any behavioural responses indicating conscious awareness of the sounds. As music was played, he gradually became able to demonstrate a level of awareness of the music evidenced by consistent and reproducible breaks in his crying and slowly moving his head towards the source of sound, smiling as he began to regulate his breathing. Boeseler (2012) states that the psychophysiological parameters, for example changes in breathing rhythm, muscle tone and heart rate, are meaningful due to the implicit intersubjective resonances, mimicries, co movements and interactional related behaviours that may occur (Boeseler 2012).

The use of music in this sensitive and attuned way repeatedly helped Gerry to reduce distress and become calm. His ability to respond to music became an integral aspect of his overall care. As one of the nurses stated, 'Music therapy promotes calmness and relaxation for Gerry even for a few minutes which facilitates the implementation of our nursing care'. When Gerry became distressed, the nursing staff would contact the music therapist to come to his bedside, play the flute and support him to calm. The nurses fed back that this was specifically beneficial before they carried out Gerry's personal care.

Gerry's consistent responses led to the formulation of an auditory regulation programme including specific CD recordings of the identified flute music and guidelines for staff to use when required as part of his 24- hour care package to help alleviate his distress. The nurses used a chart by his bedside to monitor his responses to the music and adapt the music accordingly. They recorded his behaviours as the CD played. On discharge, the CD recordings and auditory stimulation programme were sent to his ongoing care facility as part of his interdisciplinary team discharge package. This input proved continuously beneficial; staff in his ongoing care facility reported that they continued to use the CDs and requested regular updated CDs up to two years post discharge.[1]

Final thoughts

The role of the arts manager in hospital is like that of a broker, negotiating the space between service users, artists, clinical staff and hospital management. It is a world that involves developing creative initiatives and projects; but I think as artists, managers and clinicians we often start in the wrong place with arts and health work (van Roessel and Shafer 2006). I am utterly convinced that the work must always start with listening to the service user, observing, waiting and noticing. To quote a recent *New Yorker* cartoon: *We do a lot of amazing work bringing the arts to people who don't want the arts* (The New Yorker 2020). The next chapter focuses on what we might hear when we truly listen to service users.

Note

1   For more information on the music therapy service at the National Rehabilitation Hospital, Dublin see www.nrh.ie/rehabilitation-services/clinical-therapy-rehabilitation-services/music-thearpy-2/.

Further reading

The following texts explore further the ideas started in this chapter. Again, they are a guide only and independent exploration is encouraged.

Egan, G. (2018) *The skilled helper: a client-centred approach*, 2nd ed. Australia: Cengage.

Haidet, P., Jarecke, J., Yang, C., Teal, C.R., Street, R.L. and Stuckey, H. (2017) Using Jazz as a Metaphor to Teach Improvisational Communication Skills. *Healthcare (Basel)*, 5(3).

Harvey, A. (2018) *Music, evolution, and the harmony of souls*. Oxford: Oxford University Press.

Stickley, T. and Freshwater, D. (2006). The art of listening in the therapeutic relationship. *Mental Health Practice*, 9(5), 12–18, available: http://dx.doi.org/10.7748/mhp2006.02.9.5.12.c1899.

References

Ahessy, B. (2017). Songwriting with clients who have dementia: a case study. *The Arts in Psychotherapy*, 55, 23–31.

Awdish, R.L.A. and Berry, L.L. (2017). Making time to really listen to your patients. Harvard Business Review, available: https://hbr.org/2017/10/making-time-to-really-listen-to-your-patients.

Beckman, H.B. and Frankel, R.M. (1984) The effect of physician behavior on the collection of data. *Ann Intern Med*, 101(5), 692–6, available: http://dx.doi.org/10.7326/0003-4819-101-5-692.

Boeseler, K. (2012) Need-oriented, emotional communicative dialogue in music therapy with coma/apallic syndrome patients in neurological early rehabilitation. *Vegetative state: a paradigmatic problem of modern societies: Medical, ethical, legal and social perspectives on chronic disorders of consciousness*, 7–94.

Bradt, J., Dileo, C., Magill, L. and Teague, A. (2016) Music interventions for improving psychological and physical outcomes in cancer patients. *Cochrane Database of Systematic Reviews*, available: https://doi-org.proxy.lib.ul.ie/10.1002/14651858.CD006911.pub.

Bradt, J., Dileo, C. and Potvin, N. (2013a) Music for stress and anxiety reduction in coronary heart disease patients. *Cochrane Database of Systematic Reviews*, available: http://dx.doi.org/10.1002/14651858.CD006577.pub3.

Bradt, J., Dileo, C. and Minjung, S. (2013b) Music interventions for preoperative anxiety. *Cochrane Database of Systematic Reviews*, available: https://doi.org/10.1002/14651858.CD006908.pub2.

Campbell, D. (2013) Mid Staffs hospital scandal: the essential guide, *The Guardian*, available: www.theguardian.com/society/2013/feb/06/mid-staffs-hospital-scandal-guide.

Chang, H.-K., Peng, T.-C., Wang, J.-H. and Lai, H.-L. (2011) Psychophysiological responses to sedative music in patients awaiting cardiac catheterization examination: a randomized controlled trial. *Journal of Cardiovascular Nursing*, 26(5), E11–E18.

Coope, S. (2020) *MDU guide for consultants – Staying patient focused – The MDU*, available: www.themdu.com/guidance-and-advice/guides/consultant-pack/staying-patient-focused.

Edgar, A. and Pattison, S. (2006) Need humanities be so useless? Justifying the place and role of humanities as a critical resource for performance and practice *British Journal of Medical Humanities*, 32, 92–8.

Egan, G. (2018) *The skilled helper: a client-centred approach*, 2nd ed. Australia: Cengage.

El Boghdady, M. and Ewalds-Kvist, B.M. (2020) The influence of music on the surgical task performance: A systematic review. International Journal of Surgery, 73, 101–12.

Engel, G.L. (1977) The need for a new medical model: a challenge for biomedicine. *Science*, 196(4286), 129–36.

Fidler, H. and Miksza, P. (2020) Music interventions and pain: An integrative review and analysis of recent literature. Approaches: An Interdisciplinary Journal of Music Therapy, 12(1), available: https://approaches.gr.

Francis, R. (2013) *Report of the Mid Staffordshire NHS Foundation Trust public inquiry: executive summary*. The Stationary Office Limited, available: www.midstaffspublicinquiry. com/sites/default/files/report/Executive%20summary.pdf.

Garza-Villarreal, E., Pando, V., Vuust, P. and Parsons, C. (2017) Music-Induced Analgesia in Chronic Pain Conditions: A Systematic Review and Meta-Analysis. *Pain Physician*, 20, 597–610.

Garza-Villarreal, E.A., Wilson, A.D., Vase, L., Brattico, E., Barrios, F.A., Jensen, T.S., Romero-Romo, J.I. and Vuust, P. (2014) Music reduces pain and increases functional mobility in fibromyalgia. *Frontiers in Psychology*, 5, available: http://dx.doi.org/10.3389/fpsyg.2014.00090.

Haidet, P., Jarecke, J., Yang, C., Teal, C.R., Street, R.L. and Stuckey, H. (2017) Using Jazz as a Metaphor to Teach Improvisational Communication Skills. *Healthcare (Basel)*, 5(3).

Hanser, S.B. (2014) Music Therapy in Cardiac Health Care: Current Issues in Research. *Cardiology in Review*, 22(1), 37–42, doi: 10.1097/CRD.0b013e318291c5fc.

Harrison, M.B. and Chiota-McCollum, N. (2019) Education Research: An arts-based curriculum for neurology residents. *Neurology*, 92(8), e879–e883, available: http://dx.doi.org/10.1212/wnl.0000000000006961.

Ho, V. and Srivastava, S. (2019) Violins, medicine, and the art of listening. *Med Teach*, 1–2, available: https://doi.org/10.1080/0142159X.2019.1584277.

Huang, S.-T., Good, M. and Zauszniewski, J.A. (2010) The effectiveness of music in relieving pain in cancer patients: A randomized controlled trial. *International Journal of Nursing Studies*, 47(11), 1354–62, doi: 10.1016/j.ijnurstu.2010.03.008.

Huff, C. (2016) Active listening can help you as a musician, *Discmakers blog*, 7 June 2016, available: https://blog.discmakers.com/2016/06/active-listening-can-help-you-as-a-musician/.

Keatings, D., Bellchambers, H., Bujack, E., Cholowski, K., Conway, J. and Neak, P. (2002) Communication: Principal barrier to nurse-patient consumer partnerships. *International Journal of Nursing Practice*, 8, 16–22.

Lai, H.L. and Li, Y.M. (2011) The effect of music on biochemical markers and self-perceived stress among first-line nurses: a randomized controlled cross-over trial. *Journal of Advanced Nursing*, 67(11), 2414–24, available: https://doi.org/10.1111/j.1365-2648.2011.05670.x.

Lancet, T. (2014) The Francis report: a year on. *The Lancet*, 383(9917), 576, available: https://doi.org/10.1016/S0140-6736(14)60204-X.

Magee, W.L. and O'Kelly, J. (2015) Music therapy with disorders of consciousness: current evidence and emergent evidence-based practice. *Annals of the New York Academy of Sciences*, 1337(1), 256–62, doi:10.1111/nyas.12633.

Makama J.G., Ameh E.A., and Eguma, S.A. (2010) Music in the operating theatre: opinions of staff and patients of a Nigerian teaching hospital. *African Health Sciences*, 10, 386–9.

Mallett, J. and Dougherty, L. (2000) *Manual of clinical nursing procedures*, 5th ed. London: Blackwell Science.

Imhof M. and Janusik, L.A. (2006) Development and Validation of the Imhof-Janusik Listening Concepts Inventory to Measure Listening Conceptualization

Differences between Cultures. *Journal of Intercultural Communication Research*, 35(2), 79–98, available: https://doi.org/10.1080/17475750600909246.

Miller D.M. and O'Callaghan, C. (2010) Cancer Care. In D. Hanson-Abromeit and C.M. Colwell, eds., *Effective clinical practice in music therapy: medical music therapy for adults in hospital settings*. Silver Spring, MD: American Music Therapy Association, 217–308.

Mitchell, L.A., MacDonald, R.A. and Knussen, C. (2008) An investigation of the effects of music and art on pain perception. *Psychology of aesthetics, creativity and the arts*, 2(3), 162–70.

Mitchell, L.A. and MacDonald, R.A. (2006) An experimental investigation of the effects of preferred and relaxing music listening on pain perception. *Journal of Music Therapy*, 43(4), 295–316, doi: 10.1093/jmt/43.4.295.

Moss, H., Donnellan, C. and O'Neill, D. (2012) A review of qualitative methodologies used to explore patient perceptions of arts and healthcare. *Medical Humanities*, 38(2), 106–9, doi: 10.1136/medhum-2012-010196.

Moss, H., Donnellan, C. and O'Neill, D. (2015) Hospitalization and aesthetic health in older adults. *Journal of the American Medical Directors Association*, 16(2), 173.e11–173.e16, doi: 10.1136/medhum-2012-010196.

Moss, H. and O'Donoghue, J. (2019) An evaluation of workplace choir singing amongst Health Service staff in Ireland. *Health Promotion International*, 1–8, available: http://dx.doi.org/doi: 10.1093/heapro/daz044.

Moss, H. and O'Neill, D. (2014) The art of medicine: Aesthetic deprivation in clinical settings, *The Lancet*, 383(9922), 1032–3, available: http://dx.doi.org/10.1016/S0140-6736(14)60507–9.

Mowat, H., Bunniss, S., Snowden, A. and Wright, L. (2013) Listening as healthcare. *The Scottish Journal of Healthcare Chaplaincy*, 16.

Roche, R., Commins, S. and Farina, F. (2018) *Why science needs art: from historical to modern day perspectives*, 1st ed. London: Routledge.

Saarikallio S. (2012) Development and validation of the Brief Music in Mood Regulation Scale (B-MMR). *Music Perception*, 30, 97–105, available: http://dx.doi.org/10.1525/mp.2012.30.1.97.

Sakka, L.S. and Juslin, P.N. (2018) Emotion regulation with music in depressed and non-depressed individuals: goals, strategies, and mechanisms. *Music & Science*, 1, available: http://dx.doi.org/10.1177/2059204318755023.

Scruton, R. (2009) *Understanding music: philosophy and interpretation*. London: Bloomsbury.

Selle, E.W. and Silverman, M.J. (2017) A randomized feasibility study on the effects of music therapy in the form of patient-preferred live music on mood and pain in patients on a cardiovascular unit. *Arts & Health*, 9(3), 213–23, available: http://dx.doi.org/10.1080/17533015.2017.1334678.

Selle, E.W. and Silverman, M.J. (2020) Cardiovascular patients' perceptions of music therapy in the form of patient-preferred live music: Exploring service user experiences. *Nordic Journal of Music Therapy*, 29(1), 57–74, available: http://dx.doi.org/10.1080/08098131.2019.1663245.

Service, T. (2007) Joshua Bell: no ordinary busker. *The Guardian,* available: www.theguardian.com/music/tomserviceblog/2007/apr/18/joshuabell noordinarybusker.

Silverman, M.J. (2019) Music-based emotion regulation and healthy and unhealthy music use predict coping strategies in adults with substance use disorder: A cross-sectional study. *Psychology of Music,* available: http://dx.doi.org/10.1177/0305735619854529.

Silverman, M., Letwin, L. and Nuehring, L. (2016) Patient preferred live music with adult medical patients: a systematic review to determine implications for clinical practice and future research. *The Arts in Psychotherapy,* 49, 1–7, available: http://dx.doi.org/10.1016/j.aip.2016.05.004.

Spintge R. (2004) Musik in Anaesthesie und Schmerztherapie. *AINS – Anästhesiologie · Intensivmedizin · Notfallmedizin · Schmerztherapie,* 35, 243–61, available: http://dx.doi.org/10.1055/s-2000-10852-5.

Standley, J.M. (2000) Music research in medical treatment. In *Effectiveness of music therapy procedures: documentation of research and clinical practice.* Silver Spring, MD: American Music Therapy Association, 1–64.

Stickley, T. and Freshwater, D. (2006) The art of listening in the therapeutic relationship. *Mental Health Practice,* 9(5), 12–18, available: http://dx.doi.org/10.7748/mhp2006.02.9.5.12.c1899.

The New Yorker (2020) *Cartoons from the issue,* available: www.newyorker.com/cartoons/issue-cartoons.

Ullmann Y., Fodor L., Schwarzberg I., Carmi N., Ullmann A. and Ramon, Y. (2008) The sounds of music in the operating room. *Injury,* 39, 592–7.

Vaag, J., Saksvik, P.Ø., Theorell, T., Skillingstad, T. and Bjerkeset, O. (2013) Sound of well-being – choir singing as an intervention to improve well-being among employees in two Norwegian county hospitals. *Arts & Health,* 5(2), 93–102, available: http://dx.doi.org/10.1080/17533015.2012.727838.

van Roessel, P. and Shafer, A. (2006) Music, medicine, and the art of listening. *Journal for Learning through the Arts,* 2.

Warren, J.R. (2014) *Music and ethical responsibility.* Cambridge: Cambridge University Press.

Weger, H., Castle Bell, G., Minei, E.M. and Robinson, M.C. (2014) The relative effectiveness of active listening in initial interactions. *International Journal of Listening,* 28(1), 13–31, available: http://dx.doi.org/10.1080/10904018.2013.813234.

Williams, A. (2013) *The Listening Organisation: Ensuring care is person-centred in NHS Wales.* Improving Healthcare White Paper Series – No.11, Wales: 1000 Lives Plus, available: www.1000livesplus.wales.nhs.uk/.

Zengin, S., Kabul, S., Al, B., Sarcan, E., Dogan, M. and Yildirim, C. (2013) Effects of music therapy on pain and anxiety in patients undergoing port catheter placement procedure. *Complementary Therapies in Medicine,* 21(6), 689–96, available: http://dx.doi.org/10.1016/j.ctim.2013.08.017.

2 Self-expression

Telling my story

Introduction

A visit to hospital is almost universally anxiety provoking. We are outside our comfort zone and our normal environment. We are attended to by strangers, all of whom focus on the part of us that is not working well. We are worried about what will be found, and to a certain extent we come closer to facing our mortality than in everyday life. We are not in control of our environment. Often, service users have described to me the de-individualisation of institutional care. A few weeks in hospital brings a new routine of time (no longer can you stay up until 2 a.m. and sleep in until 11 a.m. if you so choose); food (no options to eat your own food, choices are often limited and of questionable quality); bed linen and so on. Friends, work and social life are put on hold. For those with longer illness and longer stay, the effects of this sterile environment are exacerbated.

The arts offer a vehicle through which to express one's individuality, reflect and potentially make sense of a frightening experience. They offer health professionals an alternative view of familiar diagnoses and the clinical environment, stopping us in our well-worn tracks to view serious illness through a new prism: that of the person who is ill. For vulnerable people with serious health issues (sometimes with very little ability to communicate verbally or in written form) the arts can offer the opportunity to narrate our story, gain a sense of control over our circumstances and find hope and beauty within the sterile, alarming environment of the healthcare institution. The arts can offer opportunities to feel less alone, to create community, and, potentially, to reduce social isolation. These are grand claims but will be explored and illustrated in this chapter.

From 2003 to 2016, I embarked on a series of projects in an acute hospital. I worked with eminent writers, visual artists, musicians, film makers, dancers, performers, composers, illustrators and photographers. All undertook different projects, including bedside arts projects, community-based recovery groups, creating original artworks and curating an arts and health themed festival. As I managed these varied projects, a common theme emerged. This was the opportunity the arts afforded people to 'tell their story' and to cope with serious illness through creative expression.

Neil's story

> I was in hospital for three weeks. Everyone was concerned with the bit of me that was ill. Physiotherapists, doctors, nurses, nursing assistants, occupational therapists. They all visited me to attend to my leg which wasn't working. Every moment of every day became a focus on my leg. Why is it not working? Testing it, testing the rest of my body, making me exercise, cleaning the wound. My working life, social life and hobbies were put on hold. I felt reduced to being just a bad leg. The rest of me felt irrelevant.

These are not new themes, and have been covered previously in several books and papers, but this chapter focuses on the role of musical narrative in coping with serious illness and making meaning out of crisis. Later chapters continue by exploring the themes of retaining identity and hope while surviving a serious illness journey and the importance of community in adapting to serious illness, recovering and making meaning out of a health crisis.

The chapter begins with an overview of narrative through the arts.

Narrative through the arts

Musicians tell stories, communicate ideas, emotions and sounds. Scientists look for quantitative evidence that music helps or makes a difference to health and well-being outcomes. This book is not concerned with proving these benefits, or with having an argument between methodological approaches to the same phenomenon. The failure to listen to the experience of people with illness described in Chapter 1 can, I believe, damage the well-being and resilience of service users. The absence of normal access to the arts in healthcare settings can deprive the person of their basic human need to be creative and express themselves (Maslow 1969; Cold 2001; Mandoki 2007; O'Connell et al. 2013; Moss and O'Neill 2014a; Moss and O'Neill 2014b; O'Neill et al. 2016).

In healthcare settings, people with serious illness, their families and the staff who care for them, all face the 'big' questions – for example, Why have I failed to revive a six year old boy? Why did I get this diagnosis? Why is my daughter one of the 4 per cent to suffer with this illness? Stories are human sense-making systems, they help us to communicate meaning, insight, perspective and articulate complexities (Bolton 2005).

Author and journalist, Sinead Gleeson describes her own journey of ill health beautifully in her memoir, *Constellations, reflections from life*:

> To escape illness or physical trauma, some turn to other forms of expression. It can feel necessary. Illness tries to diminish the sufferer, but we resist it by containing its expansion. I have never forgotten the sense of powerlessness in the face of instruction: lie down, bend forward, walk for me. I have felt it when counting backwards from ten under the stark lights of an operating theatre. Or when skin is sliced cleanly through. You are in someone else's hands. Steady, competent hands, hopefully – but the patient is never in charge. The kingdom of the sick is not a democracy.
>
> Art is about interpreting our own experience. Upon entering hospitals, or haematology wards, our identity changes. We move from artist or parent or sibling to patient, one of the sick. To commit to writing, or art, is to commit to living.
>
> (Gleeson 2019)

The biological and physical facts of a health event are the initial focus of the development of a serious illness. However, chronic illness impinges on our sense of self and in some cases requires major and sudden adaptation and adjustment in the activities of daily living. Pioneers such as Strauss and Glaser (1975) have sought to understand the meaning and experience of chronic disabling illness from both sufferers and their families' perspectives. There is a wealth of research on the role of narrative medicine (Bury 1982; Charon 2001, 2006; Morris 2008; Bramley and Matiti 2014; Glaser 1975). Central to these developments has been the idea of chronic illness as a 'disruptive event' or 'critical situation' (Bury 1982). Normally our body 'passes us by', we don't necessarily notice it when it is going well but illness disrupts this sense of normality and distorts our confidence and self-image (Williams 2000). Disruptive symptoms can affect everyday life, both at home and at work, including the giving of time to the management of symptoms or medical regimens and the socio-economic costs associated with long-term illness. Changes in body image, questions of 'why me?' or 'why now?' begin to create a complex picture of emotional and social trauma. Much of chronic illness is suffered in private, in silence, hidden away. Writer-practitioners including Michael Bury, Rita Charon and Havi Carel, among others, have worked to champion lay perspectives and experiences, to articulate the voices and concerns of those who might not otherwise have been heard (Bury 1982, 2001; Charon 2006; Carel 2018).

Stories offer a way of making human sense of dehumanised, contemporary, impersonal, regulated and unemotional organisations (Gabriel 1995). I was told a story by a manager in an industry where he was regularly required to make people redundant. He described being oblivious to the personal drama and effect on the lives of his employees until he visited a theatre production where he heard the story of redundancy from the actors playing a group of warehouse men. The manager described becoming aware, for the first time, of the devastation of redundancy from their perspective. Used wisely, the arts can play a part in education and training of clinicians, allowing the unsaid to be explored and the 'lay' voice to be the primary narrative.

Social, economic, political and familial context matters in how we cope with serious illness. For example, in Dublin in the 1970s, women did not suffer from postnatal depression, they 'got on with it' post partum, dealing with health issues without support, medical intervention or advice. In 2019 a later generation of the same family can openly acknowledge post-natal depression and seek social, medical and psychological support. A very simple argument for listening to the person's narrative when treating seriously ill people is this: the age, shock level and social background of the person receiving advice about a new diagnosis from a clinician will affect their ability to comply with medication and treatment, remember instructions and appointments and continue their exercise and social regime, which may be critical to maintaining their health and recovery. In short, illness can shatter our taken-for-granted assumptions about our bodies, ourselves and the world in which we live (Greenhalgh 1999; Charon 2001; DasGupta and Charon 2004; Strawson 2004; Wear and Aultman 2005; Houston 2006; DasGupta 2007; Morris 2008; Soundy et al. 2010; Woods 2011; Lemley and Roland 2012; Kaptein et al. 2015; Fioretti et al. 2016; Zazulak 2016; MacFarlane 2017; Moss and O'Neill 2017; Wasson 2018).

Bolton (2005) asserts that narratives are reflective tools that are essential to learning, as they penetrate our understanding more deeply than information alone. By engaging our emotions we understand more effectively, as all learning involves emotion (Bolton 2005). For service users, telling one's story may be simply having time to give an account of the traumatic experience of sudden onset of illness to key healthcare workers involved in diagnosis and treatment. For others, it may involve having time to ask questions that are pertinent to their personal circumstances, however trivial these may seem, in order to organise oneself to manage the treatment of a health problem. For others, having more time, perhaps with a therapist, to tell one's story, context and experience, can be self-affirming and may help to create order and security out of a chaotic world (Bolton 2005). In terms of coping with serious illness, we need more than ever to story and re-story our lives (Bruner 2003). As well as listening to service users (see Chapter 1) we need to also listen to ourselves, to re-story and make sense of our own experiences as clinicians or family carers (Bruner 2003).

A patient is not a person. A patient is a medicalised version of the self. A patient is a hospitalised double of the body. To become a patient is an act of transmutation, from well to sick, liberated citizen to confined inpatient. With illness, there is always a sense of a 'before' and an 'after'. The before time when everything is bright and even-keel and normal, a word that loses all meaning in the face of disease …. This may not be war, but there are two sides. The well and unwell; doctors and patients; staff and visitors. Illness gives us permission to drop everything – jobs, commitments, the tangle of repetition that is everyday life – but the price is high. Hospital requires a packed bag, but no ticket. Instead of yellow islands and turquoise shallows, there are rectangles of blankets, beds instead of sunloungers …. Is the doctor–patient exchange a dialogue, a conversation or an interrogation? Our medical narrative is contained in the clipboard hanging on the end of the bed, or in the coloured cardboard folder. We repeat our story to multiple doctors and the file swells, in different handwriting, a collaborative piece of text.

(Gleeson 2019)

Pacelli's story

Pacelli was a 65-year-old retired teacher of history and English. He enjoyed amateur dramatics and the craft of wood turning and had an active retirement pursuing these two creative activities. One day, out of the blue, Pacelli suffered a cardiac event, a heart attack, and was rushed to the emergency department for surgery. He attended the hospital Cardiac Rehabilitation programme following discharge from hospital and then signed up when he saw an advert for a hospital creative writing programme available to people who had completed the rehabilitation programme (Moss and Granier 2006). Despite going through surgery, excellent care from cardiologists and a comprehensive rehabilitation programme, Pacelli described needing to reflect and re-story his life, to reflect on the issues not covered by clinical care, namely, the sudden shock of losing his healthy body, loss of confidence, the changes to his life that happened dramatically, his fear and lack of trust in himself, his plans turned upside down in a moment, the emotional fallout of missing a major family event and facing his mortality. His poem speaks of a positive energy in starting again after a major scare.

> Beginnings: In Praise of cardiac care by Pacelli O'Rourke
> To begin with,
> All focus on the Attack,
> Dramatic
> Traumatic
> Aftermath.
> Professional brilliance in theatres and cathlabs
> Mounts the counter-attack.
> Benign wounding starts the long haul back to health.
> The beginning of a new beginning.
> Their task executed,
> Cardiac Rehab
> Reaches down with the unforced forceps of knowledge, understanding
>   and reassurance
> To plait together the damaged fibres of Confidence,
> Offering the empowering tools of
> Restoration.
> Nurturing insight into the skills of management,
> Embedding the Mighty Truth
> That life and the living can and must and will go on.
> For the Event was not the beginning of the end,
> But is
> The beginning of a new beginning.

The role of musical narrative in coping with serious illness and making meaning out of crisis

Music is used in many ways to offer insight, reflection and a new prism on the experience of living with serious illness. One's life story constantly changes, and music can play an important part in making sense of serious illness, hospital experience and individualising care. Examples include the beautiful song 'Vincent' by Don McLean reflecting on mental health issues, 'Death bed' by Powfu (a current song popular on social media aimed at young teenagers) and the classic song 'The drugs don't work' by The Verve. Other pertinent examples include Pink Floyd's 'Wish You Were Here' (one of a couple of songs by this band related to the absence of a member lost to drug addiction and mental health issues); Jackson Browne's 'Fountain of Sorrow' (loneliness); John Prine's 'Hello In There' (a moving song about ageing and loneliness) and 'I see a Darkness' by Bonnie Prince Billy, as well as larger works such as the Broadway musical 'Next to Normal'.

Music and the arts can be used in healthcare spaces to assist people to assimilate traumatic and confusing experiences and re-story their lives.

> Representing an illness in art, words or photo is an attempt to explain to ourselves what has happened, to deconstruct the world and rebuild it in our own way. Perhaps articulating a life-changing illness is part of recovery. But so is finding the kind of articulation that is specific to you. Kahlo, Grealy and Spence were lights in the dark for me, a form of guidance. A triangular constellation. To me, they showed that it was possible to live a parallel creative life, one that overshadows the patient life, nudging it off centre stage. That it was possible to have an illness but not to be the illness. They linked the private (isolated) world of the sick to the public one of creative possibility. … in taking all the pieces of the self, fractured by surgery, there is rearrangement: making wounds the source of inspiration, not the end of it.
>
> (Gleeson 2019)

Listening to personally meaningful music

Playlists of personally meaningful music are a way to connect with a person, to validate their individuality and recognise their unique personality, context and life story. The act of listening to music together can be an opportunity for reflection, dialogue and self-expression, imperative for family carers as much as service users. Playlist technology or live music performance of personally meaningful songs can be used to achieve this, but what matters is the opportunity the songs afford to listen to the person's experiences and get to know them as an individual. A colleague of mine, a pain specialist, has assimilated a playlist of songs associated with every village, town and county in his region of the health service. He works with people with long-term chronic pain and believes that the relationship he builds with the person is crucial to effectively identifying the source of their pain and assisting them to alleviate it. He asks his service users where they are from and will reference music relevant to the area or ask them about meaningful music in their lives. He does this to assist the person to trust him, to feel that he understands them. In this case, music is a simple tool to validate the individual, help them feel comfortable and learn a little about them. The universal appeal and strong personal preferences of music are used here to connect with the individual.

Music in the waiting room

Many clinicians provide music or radio in the waiting room of their clinic. This can be both a help and an irritation to service users. Carefully selected music that appeals to the majority of people attending the clinic (for example, appropriate in terms of music era, genre, volume and age) can offer a feeling of being cared for during the waiting experience. Music wisely chosen for its pace, volume and harmonic structure can ease the tense atmosphere of the room. Arguably, live music can offer even more benefit as it can be adjusted to be personally meaningful to the people present, offer positive distraction and evidence of the institution valuing the person waiting. The same consultant mentioned above has been a pioneer in testing live versus recorded music in his clinic waiting rooms. Preliminary results (in press) indicate that both types of music improved the waiting experience and the anxiety levels of service users, but live music was the most effective. In both cases, personally meaningful songs were chosen, and the creation of the music intervention was a collaborative effort between music therapist, consultant anaesthetist and service users.

Musical improvisation

Music therapists improvise with service users. They also use familiar music and songs that are important to a person in order to build a relationship – these songs provide a sense of security and comfort – as well as totally unplanned and unstructured free improvisation (Ruud 1998; Carroll 2013). Improvisatory music-making[1] affords an opportunity for free expression without using words (Gorow 2002; Sarath 2009; Higgins 2010). The inexpressible can be expressed, the unconscious sometimes finds its way into the room and there is space to express difficult feelings such as rage, sadness and frustration through music. Music has the ability to access emotional expression (one only has to think of the power of musical moments at funerals to appreciate this) and this expression can be non-verbal (DeNora 2000, 2013). Bolton (2005) points out that often we can tell our story with words but not gain insight (for example, a person fed up with colleagues who complains throughout every coffee break). A therapist can help the person reflect on the story, be a mirror to the person, reflecting some key themes and helping a person explore and make sense of experience.

Jake's story

Jake attended an open music therapy group I facilitated in an acute psychiatry ward. I often began the group by asking people what music they listen to, to open a door to conversation and relationship that was often firmly closed or stuck. In one such group, members offered song preferences and we got to know each other as we sang the chosen songs and heard what each one liked. It was nearing Christmas and the group began to sing Christmas carols, which was both enjoyable but also felt a little paradoxical as people were facing Christmas in a locked mental health facility that was far from joyful. One service user, Jake, suggested we improvise on the drums and began to play a bongo drum heavily and loudly, with a slow beat. Jake was twenty years old and had just been told by his clinical team that he would be staying in hospital for Christmas as he was not well enough to go home, despite his desire to do so. The group joined in and the beat accelerated and grew in loudness and intensity. Following this cathartic improvisation, we were able to discuss the difficulty of staying on the ward at Christmas and the frustration and anger at clinicians who held this decision-making power. The drumming had brought the unspoken feelings of frustration and sadness to the fore which opened the way for a new conversation. Jake was able to express himself without words and others connected with the feeling in the music before anyone consciously thought of the words to express their struggles. There was a strong unspoken connection through the shared tempo, pulse and rhythmic pattern in the music, which may have enabled people to share verbally following the music. The music also changed the atmosphere in the room from a pseudo-joyful carol singing session to something more authentic to the moment.

Jake's example made no difference to the length of his stay or to his medication (it is possible he left the group better able to cope with his emotions but we don't know for sure). However, this intervention contributed to the ward environment, his quality of life and, hopefully, to his coping with his illness. It is not always enough to have a potential solution or a medical treatment, sometimes a listening stance and a human approach to care is equally important. It is not that the humanities or music specifically make us more caring or more empathic but that through music the story of the person with the illness, which is so important, can be expressed.

Song writing

Song writing is a form of self-expression, present in the earliest iterations of humanity to the present day. Song writing as part of music therapy is described as the process of creating, notating and/or recording lyrics and music by the client or clients and therapist within a therapeutic relationship to address psychosocial, emotional, cognitive and communication needs of the client (Baker 2005). On surface level, listening to the words of service users through any of the arts is obvious in its power, worth and strength. I contend that music adds something special. The harmony and emotional effect of music a power to the words and an emotional intensity to the lyrics.

> To sing is to give voice to ourselves, to bring the song to life within our own bodies and to layout and interpret its verbal and musical messages

to the listener. To sing is to express and release our inner world within a safe container ... When we create a song, we also have an opportunity to hear the beauty and ugliness of our life ... The most common goals for using songs in psychotherapy are: greater self-understanding and acceptance, self-expression and the appropriate release of feelings, value and belief clarification, healthier emotional life, improved relationships with others, greater meaning and fulfillment in life, and spiritual development.

(Bruscia 2012)

Lynn's story

Lynn was a 10-year-old girl with a complex medical history who was an in-patient in a city paediatric hospital when she met Siân Brown, her music therapist. Lynn was referred to music therapy by the Occupational Therapist due to severe pain, missing a lot of school and her love of music, singing and dancing. Lynn's referral form listed Perthes Disease and hypermobility as her diagnosis. Her therapist described her as a lively, beautiful girl.

During their early sessions Lynn talked about all the old Irish songs that her Granddad played in the house and her favourite current song by Adele and the soundtrack to the film *The Greatest Showman*. She tried some percussion instruments but was resistant to any form of songwriting saying she wouldn't have the patience for writing songs. Her attention span was short, but they played some musical games together.

Lynn continued to attend weekly music therapy sessions and during the third session, the therapist found her in good spirits. Lynn chose to listen to the song *Boneless* by Steve Aoki. The therapist felt this was interesting as Lynn's illness was related to bone health. Lynn and the therapist danced together to this song and Lynn showed the therapist some new dance moves. This was fun and seemed to help develop the relationship. Soon after this, Lynn mentioned she might like to write a song and the therapist quickly agreed. As they drew a spider diagram of song ideas, Lynn talked about what she had been through with her illness over the past few years, multiple hospital visits and symptoms. The therapist listened carefully and compassionately, and Lynn took her pen and wrote 'I struggle with chronic pain.' The therapist writes:

Lynn looked at me for a reaction. Compassionately, and with steady eye contact, I repeated the line 'I struggle with chronic pain' and further replied '... that doesn't sound like fun.' She answered, 'It's no fun.' This was written down and became another line within the song. She then informed me the diagram was finished and we began to write the song at the piano. I took the chords C and E minor from a song we were previously singing that she liked and used them as I began singing 'My name is Lynn and this is my story …' I proceeded to sing the main themes from the diagram. Lynn seemed excited. Then I sang 'It's no fun, no fun, no fun' twice as a chorus. Lynn enjoyed this and joined in singing it the next time round. She started to gather some instruments and asked me to play it again. She then joined in singing the chorus and playing egg shakers and the triangle. Lynn left the session excited to tell her mum about the song.

Next week, Lynn arrived on crutches and had sore hips. She seemed tired and low in mood. She wanted to hear her song and wondered if the therapist had typed out the lyrics and chords, which she had. Lynn spent the whole session playing the song over and over again as she sang bits and played various instruments along with it. She left ten minutes early due to tiredness and pain. The therapist told her she would bring a recording device the following week so they could put her song on a CD. Lynn contributed instruments to the recording – claves, triangle, tambourine – as well as experimenting with high notes on the piano. In the last session Lynn asked to run through all the musical games they had played in previous sessions and some of the dance moves. The therapist felt she was frantically trying to fit everything in one last time. Then they sang her song and listened to the CD which Siân had brought her. She was delighted with it. As she left with her mum she turned back, waved and said one more time 'Thanks for my song Siân!'

Listen and watch online 2.1: Song by Lynn Barret age 10 and Siân Brown, Music therapist* for all audio files marked with * in this chapter, see List of online files for access details on p. ix.

Song lyrics
My name is Lynn and this is my story
On February 17th I was diagnosed with fibromyalgia and holes in
    my hips
I struggle with chronic pain
It's no fun, no fun, no fun
It's no fun, no fun, no fun
I have to go to Crumlin hospital and get x-rays and MRIs
I hate lying still in the scanner for so long
It's boring, boring and no fun
It's no fun, no fun, no fun
I'm sick of wheelchairs and splints and crutches

I'm sick of this disease
I'm sick of not being able to sleep for crying
I just wish I was free
It's no fun, no fun, no fun
It's no fun, no fun, no fun
If in 2020 they said to me I was cured of everything
I would shout out at the top of my lungs 'I'm free, I'm free, I'm free,
I'm free, I'm free, I'm free'.

It Made You

It Made You is an album of original songs written by songwriters of St.
Patrick's Mental Health Services and renowned Irish songwriter Sean
Millar. Sean worked with service users, facilitating ten weeks of collaborative songwriting workshops through which stories about life, love, loss,
strength and recovery were told. The result is a very special album of nine
original songs, written as part of the service's initiative called 'Walk in my
shoes'. The album was recorded and produced by Gavin Glass at Orphan
Recording and features the voices of Sean Millar, Gavin Glass, Jack
Lukeman, Cillian Gavin, Aoife Cullinane, Brendan Carvill, Kevin Nolan
and Paula Higgins. The project was managed and facilitated by music therapist Paula Higgins, who writes:

> The album is a celebration of the creativity that exists within each of
> us, the creativity that connects us so meaningfully to each other. We
> are incredibly proud of every person who participated in the project
> for creating such a wonderfully powerful piece of art. Central to being
> emotionally healthy is the gift of being able to find meaning in our lives.
> For many, music and the process of creating music is a central part of
> finding meaning. Connecting with our creative selves can help us over-
> come even the deepest challenges and can lift us beyond the everyday
> to experience the beauty of the arts.

Higgins facilitated group and individual therapy for people at all stages of
the mental health journey. One of her innovations was to create a music
therapy room which doubles as a music space for service users to use as they
please. The room is attractive, relaxing and inviting, a space away from the
wards and busyness of hospital. Service users can obtain a pass from their
ward manager or security office, sign themselves in and make use of this
quiet space out of hours. In itself, this simple gesture of availability of this
beautiful space reminds service users that their musical interests are part of
them, and they matter. Unlimited access to the music room gives service

users an opportunity for self-expression,, reflection or quiet listening when they need it.

Listen and watch online 2.2–2.5: It made you: The Waiting Room Track 9; It made you: Suspended animation Track 10; It made you: Moving On Track 11; It made you: None of us are angels Track 12*

Composition

Many times, the process in music therapy is more important than the product and a completed song is not the outcome. Composers in residence offer a different experience – to create new original work in response to health issues and the hospital environment. Projects in which composers have created new work in response to the experience of migraine, dementia, stroke and Parkinson's disease have been powerful, and have allowed clinicians, carers and policy makers to quite literally hear the experience of service users. Involvement and collaboration in such projects allow service users a unique way to make their voice heard. As with all music projects in hospital, however, the key is careful, skilled curation to ensure participation and collaboration is effective.

Ian's story

Ian Wilson worked as composer in residence at Tallaght University Hospital, Dublin for four years between 2010–2015. He completed three residencies, composing new works reflecting on the illnesses of older age, namely dementia, Parkinson's disease and stroke. During each residency, he engaged with people living with these illnesses, family carers and staff in the hospital (specifically geriatricians, specialist nurses, physiotherapists, speech and language therapists, occupational therapists, nursing assistants, porters, catering staff and cleaners). The composer engaged in collaboration and communication with service users throughout the development of these works, for example through open rehearsals of the work in progress and performances of part of the work at various stages of the residency. First performances of each work were for service users and occurred in the hospital before moving to the concert stage. The Irish Chamber Orchestra partnered with the hospital for this project.

These various experiences were observed and documented. The resulting composition arose from analysis of individual stories and experiences, which the artist then interwove into a coherent whole (Moss and O'Neill 2017).

In *Bewitched*, the first composition, Wilson reflected on the illness of stroke and interviewed service users and clinicians about stroke. The resulting song cycle intertwines direct text from interviews (including three service users, a consultant geriatrician, a social worker and a speech and language therapist) with songs by Doris Day which he heard in the stroke unit in the hospital. Tina was a doctor who was interviewed for this project. In the song composed from her interview, she talks candidly about how much doctors care and how they cope with the emotional burden of looking after seriously ill people. Other doctors hearing this work expressed surprise at her honesty and commented that this work allowed an openness not always possible in their culture (Moss and O'Neill 2017).

Tina's words were transformed into song lyrics:

> You carry it with you all the time.
> I remember when I was in medical school
> You were always taught you have to be objective, you have to be
>   emotionless.
> But the longer I go on,
> The more I've realized that's not what people want.
> We're human beings.
> I don't think we can do that.
> You carry it with you all the time.
> I think people are looking for empathy
> And you can't empathise with people without feeling what they're
>   feeling.
> Of course you can't get overinvolved,
> Or else you couldn't make any decisions at all.
> You'd just be swamped.
> I don't think we can do that.

Listen and watch online 2.6: Bewitched: Carry it with you by Ian Wilson*

'Therefore I am…' by Ian Wilson is a six movement instrumental work reflecting on the experience of dementia. The work is composed for violin, viola, double bass and saxophone, with the saxophone representing the person with dementia throughout the work. Wilson undertook his own research outside the care environment, reading books on the ethics and philosophy of Alzheimer care and utilising TV documentaries and online research, as well as undertaking a wide range of observation and interactions with service users, healthcare staff, family members and staff at the local dementia charity day care centre.

Movement one of the work is entitled *The Appointment* and gives an example of how the creation of this work resulted from personal reflection and experiences within the hospital.

> The Appointment attempts to convey the busy-ness of an appointment for a person with dementia. Family members are also in the room, they want to be heard and give their opinion and the doctor has to deal with them as well as with the patient. The musical situation of the saxophone is symbolic of that of the patient, not always clearly heard, sometimes overwhelmed by the others. But, when given the chance, when listened to, that line becomes stronger and more assertive.
>
> (Ian Wilson, personal communication, 2016)

Listen and watch online 2.7: The Appointment by Ian Wilson*

The final movement of the work ends with the string players leaving the stage one by one, leaving the saxophonist on his own on the stage. The haunting loneliness of the solo saxophone improvisation that ends the work evokes a strong sense of the isolation, at times, of the person with dementia.

Listen and watch online 2.8: Autumn leaves by Ian Wilson*

The result of this residency can be summarised as creation of an original artwork of high artistic quality, creating an opportunity for increased understanding and public awareness of dementia, and creation of a new composition that has an ongoing role as a tool for students to learn about dementia. This project supports the role of the arts as a qualitative research method which can contribute to illuminating and exploring the lived experience of health and illness.

> Listen and watch online 2.9: A radio feature on music and health and Wilson's work (RTE radio Culturefile) https://soundcloud.com/ soundsdoable/culture-file-music-in-tallaght

> Listen and watch online 2.10: Documentary about Ian Wilson, Composer in residence in a hospital: *A Disconnected Rhythm* https:// vimeo.com/252153107

Final thoughts

The most potent reason for bringing service user voices to the fore in health services is the emerging evidence about impact, notably improvements in quality of care (effectiveness and efficiency gains), service user and professional experiences and health outcomes (Coulter 2012). Shifts in health policy worldwide to promote service user-centred healthcare raises expectations for new types of evidence, related to service user and family experience, to be factored into decision making at clinical, organisational and policy levels. The UK National Institute for Clinical Excellence, for example, published guidelines and quality standards for patient experience, to reinforce the need to consider service user experience (O'Flynn and Staniszewska 2012). Whilst some critics argue that narratives are selective and unstable accounts, others claim that it is a sad indictment on health services that we routinely fail to ask service users about their experience (Eaton et al. 2012). Even where illness narratives are not necessarily true or authentic in an absolute sense of the word, this does not negate, devalue or impair narratives. Rather they are still arguably useful with awareness of their social and political context (Coulter et al. 2014; Lucius-Hoene et al. 2018).

This chapter has explored the role of musical narrative, the rich combination of both verbal (lyrics) and non-verbal expression, to convey stories in all their intensity, emotion, strength and power. Creative arts promote themselves as ways of expressing what cannot be conveyed in conventional language (McNiff, 2008, p. 11). The next chapter will focus on situations where music does *not* promote health and well-being.

Note

1 Musical improvisation is the creative activity of immediate ("in the moment") musical composition, which combines performance with communication of emotions and instrumental technique as well as spontaneous response to other musicians without planning or preparation (Higgins 2010).

Further Reading

Bolton, G. (2005) *Reflective practice: writing and professional development*, 2nd ed. London: Sage.

Breslin, N. (2015) *Me and my mate Jeffrey: a story of big dreams, tough realities and facing my demons head on*. Dublin: Hachette Books Ireland.

Bury, M. (1982) Chronic illness as biographical disruption. *Sociology of Health and Illness*, 4, 167–82.

Carel, H. (2018) *Illness: the cry of the flesh*, 3rd ed. Abingdon: Routledge.

Gleeson, S. (2019) *Constellations: reflections from life*. London: Picador.

References

Bolton, G. (2005) *Reflective practice: writing and professional development*, 2nd ed. London: Sage.

Bramley, L. and Matiti, M. (2014) How does it really feel to be in my shoes? Patients' experiences of compassion within nursing care and their perceptions of developing compassionate nurses. *Journal of Clinical Nursing*, 23(19–20), 2790–99, available: http://dx.doi.org/10.1111/jocn.12537.

Bruner, J.S. (2003) *Making stories: law, literature, life*. Cambridge, MA: Harvard University Press.

Bruscia, K. (2012) *Case examples of music therapy for the use of songs in psychotherapy*. Gilsum, NH: Barcelona.

Bury, M. (1982) Chronic illness as biographical disruption. *Sociology of Health and Illness*, 4, 167–82.

Bury, M. (2001) Illness narratives: fact or fiction? *Sociology of Health & Illness*, 23(3), 263–85, available: http://dx.doi.org/10.1111/1467-9566.00252.

Carel, H. (2018) *Illness: the cry of the flesh*, 3rd ed. Abingdon: Routledge.

Carroll, D. and Lefebvre, C. (2013) *Clinical improvisation techniques in music therapy: a guide for students, clinicians and educators*. Springfield, IL: Charles C. Thomas.

Charon, R. (2001) Narrative Medicine: a model for empathy, reflection, profession, and trust. *JAMA: The Journal of the American Medical Association*, 286(15), 1897–902, doi: 10.1001/jama.286.15.1897.

Charon, R. (2006) *Narrative medicine: honoring the stories of illness*. New York: Oxford University Press.

Cold, B. ed. (2001) *Aesthetics, well-being and health: essays within architecture and environmental aesthetics*. Aldershot: Ashgate.

Coulter, A. (2012) Patient engagement–what works? *Journal of Ambulatory Care Management*, 35(2), 80–89, doi: 10.1097/JAC.0b013e318249e0fd.

Coulter, A., Locock, L., Ziebland, S. and Calabrese, J. (2014) Collecting data on patient experience is not enough: they must be used to improve care. *BMJ*, 348, g2225, available: https://doi.org/10.1136/bmj.g2225.

DasGupta, S. (2007) Between stillness and story: lessons of children's illness narratives. *Pediatrics*, 119(6), e1384–91, available: https://doi.org/10.1542/peds.2006-2619.

DasGupta, S. and Charon, R. (2004) Personal illness narratives: using reflective writing to teach empathy. *Academic Medicine*, 79(4), 351–6.

DeNora, T. (2000) *Music in everyday life*. Cambridge: Cambridge University Press.

DeNora, T. (2013) *Music asylums: wellbeing through music in everyday life*. Farnham: Ashgate.

Eaton, S., Collins, A., Coulter, A., Elwyn, G., Grazin, N. and Roberts, S. (2012) Putting patients first. *BMJ*, 344, e2006, available: https://doi.org/10.1136/bmj.e2006.

Fioretti, C., Mazzocco, K., Riva, S., Oliveri, S., Masiero, M. and Pravettoni, G. (2016) Research studies on patients' illness experience using the Narrative Medicine approach: a systematic review. *BMJ*, 6, e011220.

Gabriel, Y. (1995) The unmanaged organization: stories, fantasies and subjectivity. *Organization Studies*, 16, 477–501.

Gleeson, S. (2019) *Constellations: reflections from life*. London: Picador.

Gorow, R. (2002) *Hearing and writing music: professional training for today's musician*. Gardena, CA: September Publishing.

Greenhalgh, T. (1999) Narrative based medicine: narrative based medicine in an evidence based world. *BMJ*, 318, 323–5.

Higgins, L. (2010) *Free to be musical group improvisation in music*. Lanham, MD: Rowman & Littlefield Education.

Houston, M. (2006) *The Role of Narrative in Healthcare*. Dublin: The Arts Council.

Kaptein, A.A., Meulenberg, F. and Smyth, J.M. (2015) A breath of fresh air: images of respiratory illness in novels, poems, films, music, and paintings. *Journal of Health Psychology*, 20(3), 246–58, available: https://doi.org/10.1177/1359105314566613.

Lemley, C.K. and Roland, M.W. (2012) Narrative enquiry: stories lived, stories told. In Lapan, S., Quartaroli, M. and Riemer, F., eds., *Qualitative Research: an introduction to methods and designs*. San Francisco: Jossey-Bass, 215–42.

Lucius-Hoene, G., Holmberg, C. and Meyer, T. (2018) Introduction: chances and problems of illness narratives. In Lucius-Hoene, G., Holmberg, C. and Meyer, T., eds., *Illness narratives in practice: potentials and challenges of using narratives in health-related contexts*. Oxford: Oxford University Press.

MacFarlane, A. (2017) Does Narrative Medicine Have a Place at the Frontline of Medicine? BMJ Blog. May 30, 2017, available: https://blogs.bmj.com/medical-humanities/2017/05/30/does-narrative-medicine-have-a-place-at-the-frontline-of-medicine/.

Mandoki, K. (2007) *Everyday aesthetics: prosaics, the play of culture and social identities*. London: Ashgate.

Maslow, A. (1969) *Toward a psychology of being*. New York: John Wiley & Sons.

McNiff, S. (2008) *Art-Based Research*. London: Jessica Kingsley.

Morris, D. (2008) Narrative medicines: challenge and resistance. *The Permanente Journal*, 12, 88–96.

Moss, H. and Granier, M. eds. (2006) *Patient voices: poems by patients of The Adelaide and Meath Hospital, Incorporating the National Children's Hospital, Dublin*. Dublin: Colour Books.

Moss, H. and O'Neill, D. (2014a) The aesthetic and cultural interests of patients attending an acute hospital – a phenomenological study. *Journal of Advanced Nursing*, 70(1), 121–9, available: http://dx.doi.org/10.1111/jan.12175.

Moss, H. and O'Neill, D. (2014b) The art of medicine: Aesthetic deprivation in clinical settings. *The Lancet*, 383(9922), 1032–3, available: http://dx.doi.org/10.1016/S0140-6736(14)60507-9.

Moss, H. and O'Neill, D. (2017) Narratives of health and illness: Arts-based research capturing the lived experience of dementia. *Dementia*, available: http://dx.doi.org/10.1177/1471301217736163.

O'Connell, C., Cassidy, A., O'Neill, D. and Moss, H. (2013) The Aesthetic and Cultural Pursuits of Patients with Stroke. *Journal of Stroke and Cerebrovascular Diseases*, 22(8), e404–e418, doi: 10.1016/j.jstrokecerebrovasdis.2013.04.027.

O'Flynn, N. and Staniszewska, S. (2012) Improving the experience of care for people using NHS services: summary of NICE guidance *BMJ*, 344, d6422, doi: 10.1136/bmj.d6422.

O'Neill, D., Jenkins, E., Mawhinney, R., Cosgrave, E., O'Mahony, S., Guest, C. and Moss, H. (2016) Rethinking the medical in the medical humanities. *Medical Humanities*, 42(2), 109–14, available: http://dx.doi.org/10.1136/medhum-2015–010831.

Ruud, E. (1998) *Music therapy: improvisation, communication, and culture*. Gilsum, NH: Barcelona.

Sarath, E. (2009) *Music theory through improvisation a new approach to musicianship training*. New York: Routledge.

Soundy, A., Smith, B., Cressy, F. and Webb, L. (2010) The experience of spinal cord injury: using Frank's narrative types to enhance physiotherapy undergraduates' understanding, *Physiotherapy*, 96(1), 52–8, available: https://doi.org/10.1016/j.physio.2009.06.001.

Strauss, A. and Glaser, B. (1975) *Chronic Illness and the Quality of Life*. St. Louis: Mosby.

Strawson, G. (2004) Against Narrativity. *Ratio*, 17(4), 428–52, available: https://doi.org/10.1111/j.1467-9329.2004.00264.x.

Wasson, S. (2018) Before narrative: episodic reading and representations of chronic pain. *Medical Humanities*, 44(2), 106–12, available: http://dx.doi.org/10.1136/medhum-2017–011223.

Wear, D. and Aultman, J.M. (2005) The limits of narrative: medical student resistance to confronting inequality and oppression in literature and beyond. *Medical Education*, 39(10), 1056–65, available: https://doi.org/10.1111/j.1365-2929.2005.02270.x.

Williams, S. (2000) Chronic illness as biographical disruption or biographical disruption as chronic illness? Reflections on a core concept. *Sociology of Health & Illness*, 22(1), 40–67, available: https://doi.org/10.1111/1467-9566.00191.

Woods, A. (2011) The limits of narrative: provocations for the medical humanities. *Medical Humanities*, available: http://dx.doi.org/10.1136/medhum-2011–010045.

Zazulak, J. (2016) Why narrative-based medicine is important for communicating with your older adult patients. *McMaster Optimal Aging Portal*, 18 May 2016, available: www.mcmasteroptimalaging.org/blog/detail/professionals-blog/2016/05/18/why-narrative-based-medicine-is-important-for-communicating-with-your-older-adult-patients.

3 Dissonance

When music doesn't work

This chapter takes a close look at negative aesthetics, barriers to positive musical experiences in healthcare settings (of which there are many) and indicators against music (the assumption often being that music is 'good for you', often reinforced by evangelical arts and health champions). This chapter seeks to explore when music is *not* so good for you and point to contraindications to music as part of clinical care.

The field of music, health and well-being suffers from enthusiastic practitioners who over-claim the benefits of music in healthcare. Critical literature is rare to find. There is insufficient literature about the negative effects of music or contraindications of music in healthcare. Much of the literature over-claims benefits from studies with weak methodological rigour (Moss and O'Neill 2014; Moss et al. 2015). Very few writers have focused on negative effects of cultural activities. Two notable examples exist (Kreutz and Brünger 2012; DeNora and Ansdell 2014), but critical writing in this area is relatively scarce. More often we read anecdotal reports of wonderful music programmes in hospital, with little critique of potential noise pollution, poor quality performance or lack of choice for service users. Critique is urgent in this field of work, along with standards of care and training for all musicians working in healthcare settings.

I have witnessed many poor music performances in hospital. Well-meaning volunteers who fail to offer choice of repertoire or play out of tune! Few hospitals have concrete written guidelines or directions for the aesthetic dimensions of hospital and this is arguably a neglected field (Caspari et al. 2006; Caspari et al. 2007; Caspari et al. 2011). 'If music can provide pleasure … it can also be used to inflict pain. In short, if music can liberate the human spirit, it can also be used as a mechanism of regulation and social control' (Garofalo 2011).

Berleant identified two instances of negative aesthetics: firstly, the absence of positive aesthetics (for example, blandness) and secondly, negative aesthetic experiences such as traffic noise or pollution (Saito 2017).

Anaesthetics are experiences that are dull, numbing and/or alienating, while unesthetic experiences are those that are ugly, graceless and repulsive. In health care settings we regularly observe both. Blandness, boredom and lack of creative stimulation are commonplace in nursing homes and hospitals. Noise pollution is common on hospital wards. My own research indicated that less than 50 per cent of older people in an acute hospital ward in Dublin had control over whether the radio or television was on or off and whether they had choice of what to listen to or watch (Moss et al. 2015). Mandoki introduces the concept of 'aesthetic poisoning' whereby those responsible for aesthetics only deal with perceived 'good' art (often high art) and anything less positive aesthetically is brushed under the carpet and ignored (Mandoki 2007).

In hospital we are confronted daily with mortality, disfiguration and scars. We face fear, uncertainty and discomfort. The role of the arts in assisting wayfinding and making the intangible tangible (for example, communicating a welcome or caring atmosphere) can be useful here (Moss and O'Neill 2019). However, one must be careful of the strong link between music and emotional responses which, whilst often positive, can result in distress if presented in an insensitive way (MacDonald et al. 2002; Juslin and Sloboda 2009).

Saito, in her unique work on everyday aesthetics, goes on to argue that the everyday aesthetics, such as listening to the radio, are more important in hospital and healthcare environments than access to 'high arts' such as live performances by professional musicians (Saito 2017). The majority of literature in the field of arts and health focuses on practical, active engagement with the arts rather than receptive arts (Moss et al. 2012). Of course, beauty, music and positive aesthetics are highly subjective. For example, in some African countries a deformed lower lip is a sign of beauty and tattoos are viewed as beautiful or ugly depending on context and culture (Mandoki 2007). It is possible, therefore, that the eager amateur musician who wishes to play in hospital for service users believes their music is beautiful and some people may experience it as so. There is no absolute standard to which we can refer. The context – in this case a health care setting – and current political stance are crucial in deciding what might be considered beautiful and whether investment is made in hospital aesthetics (Mandoki 2007). In my view, however, the value and appreciation of high-quality and trained musicians should hold in hospitals as it does in the concert hall, and we should not expect or allow lower standards in hospital. The provision of music in hospitals competes with utilitarian demands, and as beauty and music have no obvious use they can be undervalued by public policy makers. The importance of beauty and music lies in its absence, and it may not be noticeable to policy makers until it is not there or provided badly (De

Botton 2006; Bauman 2010; Commission for Architecture and the Built Environment 2010). In an age of financial austerity it is tempting to think of beauty, music and art as needless decorative expenses (Kieran 2005; Bauman 2010). The temptation is to cover up the unpleasant aspects of hospital (needles, bodily fluids, the spilling of food while eating) with cleanliness, hygiene and sterility accompanied by 'pleasant' music in the waiting room (Forsey and Aagaard-Mogensen 2019). People with serious illnesses often describe people avoiding them, not knowing what to say. How then, do we approach musical engagement if we do not allow the dissonance of human experience to be heard?

There are several myths in existence regarding the benefit of music in hospitals.

Myth 1: Music is good for everyone

Music in public spaces (whether healthcare spaces, shops, restaurants or other public environments) can be irritating and annoying. Noise pollution is a problem in healthcare spaces and research on the aesthetics of hospital finds lack of provision for *choosing* different kinds of aesthetic input as the area of most dissatisfaction for service users (Lawson and Phiri 2003; Caspari et al. 2006; Caspari et al. 2007; O'Connell et al. 2013; Moss et al. 2015; Caspari et al. 2018). Personal associations with music can create sadness, upset and distress as often as joy and happiness. Music is not a panacea. Skilful curation is required to ensure that the benefits available from engagement in music are carefully matched to service users who need this intervention. The problem with this myth is that any music will do – good, bad or indifferent. Many healthcare managers make the mistake of investing in a pilot project, or short-term initiative, but are reluctant to resource sustained music projects and view live music input as 'the icing on the cake', a trivial, frothy extra to the healthcare environment and the first thing that can be cut when budgets are tightened. A more nuanced conversation is needed to determine what music, in which situations, for whom, will be of real benefit. An acknowledgement that music can benefit and harm in equal measure is a starting point for a deeper critique of when and how music should be used in hospital. After all, as far back as Plato's *Republic*, Socrates cast doubt on the notion of a self-contained aesthetic experience, saying, 'As if music and poetry were only play and did no harm at all' (Ross 2014).

Myth 2: Music makes you a morally better person

Engagement in music doesn't make you a 'better' person despite the overreaching claims of some of my colleagues. Radovan Karadzic, for example, published eight books of poetry and won several literary awards whilst being responsible for the crime of genocide, causing the Srebrenica massacre which left 8,000 men dead. Hitler was an artist, earning money selling his watercolours and later an avid collector whose passion turned into the most brutal art theft. He funded a number of major cultural institutions in Germany during his reign of terror.

The simple stories in this book, of people expressing themselves and communicating through music, are an antidote to the over enthusiastic claims that music is somehow 'good for you' or makes you a 'better' person. We need to move beyond the idea that access to the arts will always improve a person, and explore why music matters, and has always mattered, throughout time and cultures, as part of healing rituals and well-being activities (Ansdell 2014). This is more of a qualitative enquiry than a quantitative one.

Similarly, claims that arts engagement will make doctors more caring and empathic are dubious; the field of medical/health humanities focuses on engagement with the arts to explore what it is to be human. Whilst this alternative view of illness and service user experience is welcome, claims that the arts improve empathy skills are as yet unproven. This claim also implies that clinicians and scientists are generally lacking humanity and empathy, a claim that is over-generalised and offensive to the many skilled and caring clinicians I have met in the course of my work.

Studying the humanities is valuable, but not always in the way some medical humanities scholars claim, such as causing 'remedial humanisation' or making doctors into better people (Stempsey 1999; Shapiro and Rucker 2003; O'Neill et al. 2016; Moss and O'Neill 2012; Koschorke 2018). An over focus on 'highbrow' literature in medical humanities ignores the learning (and fun) to be gained from other branches of the humanities (Crawford 2015; Crawford et al. 2020; O'Neill et al. 2020).

Myth 3: Music therapy is a new age, hippie therapy

In countries where music therapy is not a regulated clinical profession (the majority of European countries for example), music therapists struggle to be taken seriously and accepted as members of the clinical team. Regulation of the profession as a clinical profession, alongside Speech and Language Therapy, Occupational Therapy and Physiotherapy is important in protecting service users from unsafe, unqualified rogue traders as well as recognising the evidence-base of this well-established profession. For example, several systematic reviews document the health benefits of music, including Cochrane reviews and Lee's meta-analysis of 96 randomised control trials of music and pain (Bradt et al. 2016; Bradt et al. 2013a; Bradt et al. 2013b; Lee 2016; Magee et al. 2017; Bradt and Teague 2018). Outcomes include statistically significant effects in decreasing pain, emotional distress, medication intake, heart rate, blood pressure and respiration rate. There is good evidence that music has the potential to be a useful non-pharmacological intervention in the management of issues such as post-surgery pain relief, sedation in children and pre surgery anxiety, we well as being a supportive activity for people with cancer, adolescents and those in the mental healthcare environment (Daykin et al. 2008a; 2008b; 2018; Fancourt and Finn 2019; Daykin 2020). Indeed, a recent WHO report on arts and health, which represents the largest scoping review of the literature to date, concludes that there is significant evidence of benefit in key areas of healthcare, albeit with documented limitations (Fancourt and Finn 2019).

Myth 4: Sure it's great for them to have a bit of music …

In some healthcare facilities live music is appreciated as an environment enhancer, but the quality of the engagement is not considered. Clinical staff and managers are quick to accept offers from well-meaning amateurs, whether or not the standard of music is high. Music is a powerful and effective intervention and highly qualified, skilled musicians should always be engaged. A lack of appreciation of high-quality music is a societal issue and not reserved for healthcare services. If society and our government do not fund high quality music education accessible to all, then standards fall and this affects all areas of society, including healthcare settings. As the arts manager in hospital, I programmed live classical music, traditional Irish sessions, choir performances, composers in residence, music participation classes in the hospital school, music therapy sessions and more. My bottom line was that whoever the musician was, and no matter which approach the person was bringing to music in healthcare settings, they had to have musical skills of the highest standard.

When music doesn't work

A hospital is a petri dish of anxiety. Any aesthetic enrichment undertaken in a hospital must serve a function – to address a clinical need or system problem. Simple changes using colour, art, music and video imagery can improve the experience for service users and staff by creating a reassuring, safe environment whereby people can relax, receive a more successful investigation, build positive clinical engagement and hopefully improve clinical outcomes. However, first we must explore the many negative aesthetic experiences in hospital and when music doesn't work.

Music can be damaging and unhelpful in healthcare settings. I have seen many instances where control and choice are denied and people are forced to listen to music (both live and recorded). The quality may be poor also, which is problematic, and the choice of music is weak. Catherine Tate humorously demonstrated this issue in her interview with Graham Norton on singing in a nursing home and the creation of her famous comedy character 'Nan'.

Listen and watch 3.1: Catherine Tate interview www.youtube.com/watch?v=LQco8BM1DuQ

I have identified eight instances when music is contraindicated in healthcare spaces. In all cases, it is important to note that the solution to all these problems is qualified, thoughtful, sensitive, skilled music professionals responsible for music facilitation in health care spaces.

1. *When auditory regulation is indicated*

Neonatal units and rehabilitation units for people with disorders of consciousness (PDOC) are specialised areas where music can be a necessary stimulation but can also cause distress if over-used or too loud. (See Chapter 1 Case study of Gerry at the National Rehabilitation Hospital for more information about this aspect of music-making in hospital). Expert intervention is needed for music to work well (as indicated in these 'Listen and watch' examples).

Listen and watch 3.2: Noise: The need to reduce noise in a Neonatal Intensive Care Unit www.youtube.com/watch?v=ymgFpM2t70k

Listen and watch 3.3: Music Therapy programme for premature babies www.youtube.com/watch?v=4qjx2BrrQJg

2. *When the person doesn't want music*

It seems too obvious to state choice and preference as a requirement for music in healthcare spaces but unfortunately there are too many cases where music is imposed upon unsuspecting service users who cannot escape musical intervention.

Sally's story

Sally was with her son in a paediatric ward in an acute hospital. He was 15 and had gone through serious surgery and was in pain. A musician from a respected organisation which trains musicians to work in healthcare settings visited the ward and began to play his guitar and sing at the end of this boy's bed. Sally reported that neither he, nor his mother, wanted the music and were not asked. She was so taken aback she didn't challenge the musician, neither did staff, who perceived him to be 'wonderful'. The boy was in so much pain he could not engage in any way. She said she just wanted him to go away, as did her son. Sally described another hospital stay where a local choir came to the ward to sing Christmas carols. They sang off key and with poor quality. She again felt imposed upon and offended.

Jeff's story

Jeff reported several times when he was in hospital and a local choir would come and sing carols. Each choir was different, but all were amateur, not particularly good and felt to him like noise pollution. Christmas time brought an influx of carol singers to the ward. 'If I hear one more bloody carol …'. The people singing arguably got more from the feel good factor of helping others than the service users. As a manager of music programmes in hospital there was always a flurry of local choirs and musicians wanting to perform in the week before Christmas. However, few wanted to visit on Christmas day itself or in the depressing months of early January.

It is critical that any music brought into hospital (whether receptive or participative, live or recorded) is provided only to people who want to listen and that the choice to stop listening or leave the environment is available to everyone in the environment. How do you leave a performance if you cannot move independently? I made a point of checking in at every music performance with people who needed assistance to move and those who could not express themselves easily verbally, in case they wished to leave.

3. *When the quality is poor*

Many hospitals have consulted me on music programmes, looking to bring in students, volunteers or children to play for residents. Whilst this can be excellent, it can also be piecemeal and variable. Too often, a hospital manager or nursing home manager satisfies themselves that they have ticked the 'music provision box' by bringing in Mary, a retired piano teacher who lives down the road, to play a few songs on a Friday morning. This is the equivalent of providing a retired sports coach from a local gym rather than a fully qualified physiotherapist. For sure, the gym trainer can do some really useful work, but the residents also deserve specialist input and overall programme direction from a professional qualified to support their physical health needs with clinical awareness and skills. The issue of payment always arises. Why do health service personnel expect musicians to work free or on minimal pay? I have lost count of the number of times I have been asked to provide skilful music sessions for people with serious illness for a 'pilot' of four sessions (to see if it 'works') one morning a week. Would they provide a dental care pilot in such as way? Musicians are seen as a disposable trifle and are not afforded the professionalism they deserve. Quality is key (Moss and O'Neill 2009).

4. When it is all about do-gooders

In order to train as a music therapist, I underwent a gruelling third interview with a psychologist to determine my motivation to be a music therapist. Was I just a do-gooder? Making myself feel better by helping? The term 'inspiration porn' is well documented to refer to the practice of assigning special status to people with disabilities. Coined by Stella Young, it challenges the condescending and patronising attitude that normal activity by people with disabilities is somehow inspirational and amazing (Young 2014; Grue 2016). In music research, the three adjectives used most frequently to describe musicians with disabilities are amazing, inspiring, and awesome (Young 2014; Darrow and Hairston 2016).

Why are we providing music? Why do we wish to attend a healthcare facility and play our music for clients? Is this for our own benefit or clients? As musicians, we need to be honest and self-aware, to recognise our own needs which are being met by volunteering or performing in healthcare settings.

5. When there is no assessment of need

Receptive, participative and therapeutic music is often provided without assessing the need, the desire of participants and the benefit. I always advise supervisees never to work with someone unless you know why you are doing so. When receivers are not consulted or involved in the planning of the music input, it almost always loses value.

Cindy's story

Cindy managed a hospital music programme. An arts council funding initiative allowed a composer and story teller to work in her local area and they approached the hospital wishing to work in a neonatal unit, observe what happens and write a song based on the experience. The team at the hospital were concerned. It seemed a totally inappropriate request and the artists did not demonstrate a careful thinking out of the idea and had no experience in such a clinical area prior to designing the project. Cindy felt concerned that service users (parents and their fragile babies) were being viewed as 'subject matter' for an artistic composition. Cindy tried to facilitate these artists, nonetheless, by offering a less sensitive area of the hospital in which to work. For example, they discussed working with the catering department and exploring a song around the nourishment of service users. The artists did not like this idea. Eventually the artists and the hospital representatives settled on a workable solution. It was agreed that the artists would work with the hospital choir and write a song about the choir. Once the project was over, the musical director of the choir commented that she did not think the composed song was very high quality. Cindy herself found that the song did not seem to connect with choir members. During the process, the choir had been excited as the storyteller engaged with them. They talked about the history of the work song and how this new song could be an equivalent modern-day work song. They met the storyteller but never met the composer during the whole process! Cindy was left with concerns about the quality of the music and the lack of connection between the musician and hospital staff. Perhaps the most interesting conclusion of this project is that there is nowhere where we can talk about such failed projects. Musicians, researchers and managers tend to report the good news stories of music in health contexts, never the times it goes wrong, is injurious or falls short of being helpful.

6. When music is used to control

Music is used to control, reinforce social division and preserve the power of those with higher status and control (Daykin 2020). In Guantánamo Bay detention centre, music was used to torture by playing music that was too loud, repetitive or offensive to the prisoner's culture, or to taunt prisoners about people they loved at home (Garofalo 2011). During the Holocaust, musicians in the Belzec concentration camp were forced to play a popular German song, 'Es geht alles vorüber, es geht alles vorbei' (Everything passes, everything goes by), to 'greet' the transports as they arrived. In these cases, music was a weapon of war (Stafford Smith 2008).

Music often has a prominent role in constructing cultural identities and demarcating political and social groupings (Folkestad 2002). Folk music claims territories and culture, for example music therapists in Northern Ireland attest to the sensitivity of music choices to avoid exclusion or insult (Shekhovtsov 2013). Similarly, songs at football matches and in adolescence are used to promote identification with a group. Musical groupings can alienate the 'other', by playing politically or culturally insensitive songs (Attali 1985; Warren 2014).

It is important to note that it is how music is used that creates the torture and humiliation, not the music itself. Likewise, in a hospital setting, the insensitive use of music can separate, alienate or cause injury (Shekhovtsov 2013). We can never hope to know, or anticipate, the effect that music will have on people in hospital – people who are vulnerable or have heightened emotion due to the stress of major illness or diagnosis. That is why a suitably trained clinical professional is required to select music sensitively and, more importantly, to be able to support people who have an unexpected or unusually strong reaction to music (Gabrielsson 2011). The social impact of music cannot be underestimated, in both positive and negative associations. For example, the British Union of Fascists, formed in 1932, gradually introduced musical signifiers of their regime. An anthem was chosen, and only British and Fascist music could be played by members. Eventually the organisation set up BUF choirs and even developed its own orchestra in 1934. Music was not only part of the BUF's socialising, but became an integral part of its public persona, reinforcing their views on racial superiority (Macklin 2013; Shaffer 2013; Shekhovtsov 2013)

7. When clinicians are not engaged

The engagement of clinicians is crucial in effecting positive change in the aesthetic environment of healthcare spaces. I have witnessed artists with wildly unrealistic expectations about what can be achieved in health settings who have not consulted clinicians and service users about potential projects. I have seen seasoned arts therapists create distance and mistrust by being unwilling to adapt their service to meet the needs of clinicians and managers. Ongoing communication, co-creation of services and discussion is vital for successful arts projects to flourish in healthcare spaces. The nuances of successful interdisciplinary collaboration is perfectly described by Fitzgerald and Callard (2015). Similarly, family carers are crucial partners in delivering quality services to people who need support. Family carers are the largest cohort of healthcare workers in most countries, yet attention to their needs and supports are relatively under researched. In my experience, music interventions, activities and engagements are often mis-targeted when clinicians and family carers are not consulted and involved.

8. When people need silence

In hospital, silence is a rare phenomenon. The emergency, urgency and communication of essentials leaves little space for silence. Wards shared by four or six people further reduce the possibility of silence. Silence in consultations is rare, silence makes many people feel uncomfortable and is often broken to avoid awkwardness or anxiety. Silence is defined as the absence of sound (Hornby 1995) and often associated with nothingness or death. Sound, on the other hand, is associated with life and activity. Our attempts to control our lives lead us to believe we should be able to control noise around us, and thus unwanted noise can increase anxiety in hospital. Music can be an extra noise, an unwanted sound.

There are many instances in hospital when silence is desirable. Hospitals are by their nature busy, bustling, noisy environments, Machines, monitors, large numbers of staff, trolleys and dinner trays, family visitors, phones, sounds of pain and distress, emergency crash noise. Hospitals are rarely quiet, even at night. Noise is described as 'unwanted sound' by the World Health Organisation (Berglund et al. 1999). More than half European citizens live in noisy surroundings, a third live with noise that disturbs sleep. Scientific approaches measure noise and levels of sound where physiological damage is done to the ear. However, there is no measurable amount of sound that is intrinsically bothersome. Our cultural norms and expectations affect this perception of noise (Warren 2014). Hospitals have largely been accepted as noisy atmospheres with noise disturbance known to be detrimental; studies in adult patients have linked excessive noise to sleep disturbance and increased blood pressure, heart rate, and stress (Montague et al. 2009). Silence is important in hospitals and when curating musical experiences we can also be advocates for no music and for quiet spaces.

Silence can be a rarity in human interaction, and particularly within busy health care settings. Silence can be a resting place for service users, a time when reflection can take place. But it can also be difficult to tolerate. While silence may encourage a service user to talk, it might also incite the practitioner to interject and fill what can feel like an uncomfortable empty space. Allowing silence in a healthcare institution is challenging and provides a completely different experience for the service user. Mozart is famously attributed as saying 'Music is not the notes, it is the silence between them'. And as Will Rogers said 'Never miss a good chance to shut up' (Frothingham 2013). Samuel Beckett (1906–1989) explored silence, absence and unknowing relentlessly during his career.

> Beckett often spoke about throwing away all intellectual solutions and moving away from the destructive need to dominate life ... perhaps humanities shift the territory of bioethics from the certainty of the empirical and rational world to the uncertainty, ambiguity and indeterminacy of the artistic.
>
> (Chambon and Irving 2003)

Flower (2001) highlights three experiences of silence in a music therapy setting: Silence within the client (awareness, identity, separateness), silence within the therapist (digest, think about, listen), and silence within the room (ability for both parties to tolerate and create silences). Profound insights may also be realised in silence when it is experienced as a place of rest, a place of reflection and an active agent of change (Sutton 2002).

A recent oncology study demonstrated that where the oncologist's communication included acknowledging, exploring, empathic and supportive statements, and attentive silence, the result was better information recognition (Visser et al. 2019). Part of listening to people tell their story is allowing people to be silent.

> The Buddhist monks think of silence as a form of space – internal space, space inside you and the space made in a room without any sound.
>
> (Ferber 2004)

Whether silence is a time of calm and reflection or intolerable and anxious, it is certain that silence is rare in hospitals, as reflected in Gleeson's description of her own experience.

> Trolley-trundle and siren-blare. I'm on lates this week. Whirr-blink of machines. Food trays rattling. Nuuu-rrsse! The three notes the blood pressure pump sings on completion. Pinging of patient call bells. Squeak of sensible footwear. The pneumatic door hinge opening and closing like bellows. The ghostly exhalations of those who took their last breath here. Hospitals are rarely silent.
>
> (Gleeson, 2019)

There may be times, as a music professional in a hospital, when we need to speak out about sound, noise and silence and recommend less rather than more sound. In my career I became an advocate for the creation of quiet spaces in hospital so that staff and service users could go to escape the noise and stress of ward life. A natural ally in both services was the pastoral care team whose prayer and meditation spaces are designed for this very purpose.

Recommendations

Whilst beauty and aesthetics are often reported and celebrated within healthcare settings (the internet is awash with 'beautiful hospital design' examples), ugliness is rarely written about, reported or considered. Books on negative aesthetics, noise pollution or potential negative aspects of music are relatively rare (Sibley 2001; Stecker 2006). A recent paper on the link between music listening and drug addiction is interesting in that it reports how drug taking enhances music listening experiences (Dingle et al. 2015). This opens a rare space for debate around the messier aspects of music, health and illness. Opportunities to discuss when music has not worked in hospital are difficult to find.

While we continue to navigate the journey between evidence and subjective experience, I propose some simple changes to improve the hospital atmosphere using music:

a) Carefully considered music in the waiting room. Either live or recorded music, carefully chosen and curated. The aim of this music is to communicate concern for the waiting experience and create a calm, secure environment. Rhythmically and tonally grounded music works best in this environment, not too loud or intrusive, most likely instrumental. Where possible consult widely as to which music to include and offer choice of volume, playlists and silence.

b) Listening pods with playlists. Service users can plug their headphones into a wall mounted music system in the waiting room, to listen to a playlist designed to support them. These may be songs of hope for those dealing with serious diagnoses, songs for relaxation and mindfulness with music.

c) Music therapy referrals for service users who receive complex diagnoses or undergo stressful tests. Music therapists can work alongside clinicians to enable service users to relax and engage in tests and procedure (reducing need for sedative drugs for example). For those coping with major stress, a music therapist can offer a supportive space for the person to process bad news or difficult experiences, to learn relaxation exercises and develop playlists targeted to cope with health issues.

d) Live music performance. This can lift the atmosphere of hospital, communicate care and value for the person receiving care (you have bothered to bring in musicians for me?!) and provide shared enjoyable activity for family members, service users and staff. However, always programme high quality performances, be prepared to pay for the quality and again consult and curate carefully.

e) Music as distraction. Offer opportunities for music to distract from anxiety and pain. For example, a musician working with children and babies alongside phlebotomists taking blood; live music during unpleasant procedures in Emergency departments and outpatient clinics; recorded music to support people with dementia while they wait for medical appointments and music as part of labour and perinatal mental health.

f) Skilful use of music in sensitive clinical areas. Engage a music therapist to advise on musical input in areas such as intensive care units, wards for people with disorders of consciousness and neonatal units. There is ample evidence of benefit, but music should be curated carefully and gently so as not to overstimulate or cause distress.

Final thoughts: Does music matter?

Nearly everyone listens to music at some stage of their life and music plays a key role in individualising healthcare experiences. One of the most universal questions that exists is 'What music do you like?'

I am not sure, however, that we can prove entirely by statistics or quantitative evidence that musical care and support matters or makes a difference in hospital settings. It is an ongoing question to debate whether music provided in hospitals makes a tangible difference and if so, how and when. 'Are the arts merely window dressing or institutional vanity distracting us from the real concerns of service users? Do they take money and resources away from more deserving areas? Do the arts actually make a difference? Do they merely pander to the preferences of a select and intellectual elite?' (Gallagher 2007) Answers to these questions are often subjective and personal but the more we can prove generalisable benefits the better. For example, ground-breaking work proved for the first time that listening to one's favourite music in the acute phase of stroke makes a marked difference to a range of recovery variables (Sarkamo et al. 2008). Evidence of benefit is highest for people with dementia and stroke, and work on the rehabilitative effects of music-based interventions in several neurological diseases, is advanced (Sihvonen et al. 2017). Magee's work on the benefit of music therapy for people with acquired brain damage has made huge strides in the evidence base for music as a treatment in this clinical field (Magee and O'Kelly 2015; Magee et al. 2017; Magee 2018). In my work, the evidential gains have been more subtle, but nonetheless I have witnessed day after day some exceptional examples of the power of music to effect change in communication (verbal and non-verbal), self-expression, quality of life, perception of pain and anxiety, and motivation. This brief note from a consultant anaesthetist demonstrates the potential of music in hospital care:

> I had a 70-year-old woman at the pain clinic on Friday who I know well. I left my speaker in the car that morning by error. Usually I play music in the waiting area. There were two others in the room with her. This lady is very depressed. We have a good relationship and I do injections for her. She always talks about suicide and she wants to die. Two of her adult children died by suicide/OD related to drugs. She spends a lot of time in the psychiatry unit. When she in came in the room I asked her

to listen to a song with me from my phone. I played "A woman's heart" from Eleanor McEvoy from a playlist on my phone. I then played "I will always be there for you" by Jesse Glynne. I said I would arrange an injection for her. Nothing else said. She hugged me and cried.

It is possible that care and concern about music, art and design reflects a thinking beyond the efficiency and statistics of healthcare to include a care and concern for the humans receiving this care. We will also never find a consensus about what sort of music will 'work' in healthcare and the only solution I have found is to personalise music to the individual in hospital rather than offer blanket solutions that will irritate some and please others. Personalised, individualised music-making is key – everyone likes different music, everyone has preference for silence, music, background noise, TV or nothing. It has to be a personal intervention based on service user preference and need.

This chapter explored the myths surrounding music in hospital, when it is contraindicated in clinical contexts and recommended appropriate usage. The next chapter will present some compelling international examples of how music can help in hospital.

Further Reading

Juslin P. and Sloboda J. (2009) *Music and emotion: theory and research*. Oxford: Oxford University Press.

Mandoki, K. (2007) *Everyday aesthetics: prosaics, the play of culture and social identities*. London: Ashgate.

Moss, H. and O'Neill, D. (2014) The art of medicine: Aesthetic deprivation in clinical settings. *The Lancet*, 383(9922), 1032–3, available: https://doi.org/10.1016/S0140-6736(14)60507-9.

Saito, Y. (2017) *Aesthetics of the familiar everyday life and world-making*. Oxford: Oxford University Press.

Shaffer, R. (2013) The soundtrack of neo-fascism: youth and music in the National Front. *Patterns of Prejudice*, 47(4–5), 458–82, available: https://doi.org/10.1080/0031322X.2013.842289.

References

Ansdell, G. (2014) *How music helps in music therapy and everyday life*. Farnham: Ashgate.

Attali, J. (1985) *Noise: the political economy of music*. Minneapolis: University of Minnesota Press.

Bauman, I. (2010) *Beauty, localism and deprivation*. London: Commission for Architecture and the Built Environment.

Berglund, B., Lindvall, T. and Schwela, D. (1999) *Guidelines for Community Noise*. Geneva: World Health Organisation, available: www.who.int/docstore/peh/noise/Comnoise-1.pdf.

Bradt, J., Dileo, C. and Potvin, N. (2013a) Music for stress and anxiety reduction in coronary heart disease patients. *Cochrane Database of Systematic Reviews*, available: http://dx.doi.org/10.1002/14651858.CD006577.pub3.

Bradt, J., Dileo, C. and Minjung, S. (2013b) Music interventions for preoperative anxiety. *Cochrane Database of Systematic Reviews*, available: https://doi.org/10.1002/14651858.CD006908.pub2.

Bradt, J., Dileo, C., Magill, L. and Teague, A. (2016) Music interventions for improving psychological and physical outcomes in cancer patients. *Cochrane Database of Systematic Reviews*, available: https://doi-org.proxy.lib.ul.ie/10.1002/14651858.CD006911.pub.

Bradt, J. and Teague, A. (2018) Music interventions for dental anxiety. *Oral Diseases*, 24(3), 300–306, available: http://dx.doi.org/10.1111/odi.12615.

Caspari, S., Eriksson, K. and Naden, D. (2006) The aesthetic dimension in hospital – an investigation into strategic plans. *International Journal of Nursing Studies*, 43, 851–9.

Caspari, S., Eriksson, K. and Naden, D. (2007) Why not ask the patient? An evaluation of the aesthetic surroundings in hospitals by patients. *Quality Management in Health Care*, 16(3), 280–92.

Caspari, S., Eriksson, K. and Naden, D. (2011) The importance of aesthetic surroundings: a study interviewing experts within different aesthetic fields. *Scandinavian Journal of Caring Sciences*, 25(1), 134–42.

Caspari, S., Råholm, M.B., Sæteren, B., Rehnsfeldt, A., Lillestø, B., Lohne, V., Slettebø, Å., Heggestad, A.K.T., Høy, B., Lindwall, L. and Nåden, D. (2018) Tension between freedom and dependence—a challenge for residents who live in nursing homes. *Journal of Clinical Nursing*, 27(21–22), 4119–27, available: http://dx.doi.org/10.1111/jocn.14561.

Chambon, A. and Irving, A. (2003) 'They give reason a responsibility which it simply can't bear': ethics, care of the self and caring knowledge, *Journal of Medical Humanities*, 24, 265–78.

Commission for Architecture and the Built Environment (2010) *People and places: Public attitudes to beauty*. London: Commission for Architecture and the Built Environment.

Crawford, P. (2015) *Health humanities*. Basingstoke: Palgrave Macmillan.

Crawford P. and Brown, B. and Charise, A. eds. (2020) *The Routledge Companion to Health Humanities*. Abingdon: Routledge.

Darrow, A.A. and Hairston, M. (2016) Inspiration porn: a qualitative analysis of comments on musicians with disabilities found on international youtube posts. in Belgrave, M., ed., *Proceedings of the 21st International Seminar of the ISME Commission on Special Music Education and Music Therapy*. Drake Music Edinburgh and Edinburgh University, Edinburgh, 23–26 July.

Daykin, N. (2020) *Arts, health and well-being: a critical perspective on research, policy and practice*. Abingdon: Routledge.

Daykin, N., Byrne, E., Soteriou, T. and O'Connor, S. (2008a) Review: The Impact of art, design and environment in mental healthcare: a systematic review of the literature. *The Journal of the Royal Society for the Promotion of Health*, 128(2), 85–94.

Daykin, N., Mansfield, L., Meads, C., Julier, G., Tomlinson, A., Payne, A., Grigsby, D., Lane, J., D'Innocenzo, G., Burnett, A., Kay, T., Dolan, P., Stefano, T. and Victor, C. (2018) What works for wellbeing? A systematic review of wellbeing outcomes for music and singing in adults. *Perspectives in Public Health*, 138(1), 39–46.

Daykin, N., Orme, J., Evans, D., Salmon, D., McEachran, M. and Brain, S. (2008b) The impact of participation in performing arts on adolescent health and behaviour: a systematic review of the literature. *Journal of Health Psychology*, 13(2), 251–64.

De Botton, A. (2006) *The architecture of happiness*. London: Penguin Books.

DeNora T. and Ansdell G. (2014) What can't music do? *Psychology of Well-Being: Theory, Research and Practice* 4, available: http://dx.doi.org/doi:10.1186/s13612-014-0023-6.

Dingle, G.A., Kelly, P.J., Flynn, L.M. and Baker, F.A. (2015) The influence of music on emotions and cravings in clients in addiction treatment: A study of two clinical samples. *The Arts in Psychotherapy*, 45, 18–25, available: https://doi.org/10.1016/j.aip.2015.05.005.

Fancourt, D. and Finn, S. (2019) *What is the evidence on the role of the arts in improving health and well-being? A scoping review*. World Health Organisation, available: www.euro.who.int/en/publications/abstracts/what-is-the-evidence-on-the-role-of-the-arts-in-improving-health-and-well-being-a-scoping-review-2019.

Ferber, S.G. (2004) Some developmental facets of silence: a case-study of a struggle to have a proximity figure. *British Journal of Psychotherapy*, 20(3), 315–32, available: https://doi.org/10.1111/j.1752-0118.2004.tb00146.x.

Fitzgerald, D. and Callard, F. (2015) *Rethinking interdisciplinarity across the social sciences and neurosciences*. Basingstoke: Palgrave Macmillan.

Flower, C. (2001) The spaces between the notes: Silence in music therapy. in *APMT/BSMT Annual Conference Proceedings*.

Folkestad, G. (2002) National identity and music. In MacDonald R., Hargreaves J. and Miell D., eds., *Musical identities*. Oxford: Oxford University Press, 151–62.

Forsey, J. and Aagaard-Mogensen, L. eds. (2019) *On the ugly: aesthetic exchanges*. Newcastle upon Tyne: Cambridge Scholars.

Frothingham, R.S. (2013) *The words and wisdom of Will Rogers: letters, speeches and quotes*. CreateSpace Independent Publishing Platform.

Gabrielsson, A. (2011) *Strong experiences with music*. Oxford: Oxford University Press.

Gallagher, A. (2007) The role of the arts in mental health nursing. *Journal of Psychiatric and Mental Health Nursing*, 14(4), 424–9.

Garofalo, D. (2011) Politics, mediation, social context and public use. In Juslin, P.N. and Sloboda, J.A., eds., *Handbook of music and emotion: theory, research, applications*. Oxford: Oxford University Press, 725–54.

Gleeson, S. (2019) *Constellations: reflections from life*. London: Picador.

Grue, J. (2016) 'The problem with inspiration porn: a tentative definition and a provisional critique', *Disability & Society*, 31(6), 838–49, available: http://dx.doi.org/10.1080/09687599.2016.1205473.

Hornby, A.S. (1995) *Oxford Advanced Learner's Dictionary of Current English*, 5th ed. Jonathan Crowther, ed. Oxford: Oxford University Press.

Juslin P. and Sloboda J. (2009) *Music and emotion: theory and research*. Oxford: Oxford University Press.

Kieran, M. (2005) Value of art. In Gaut, B. and McIver Lopes, D., eds., *The Routledge companion to aesthetics*, 2nd ed. Abingdon: Routledge, 293–307.

Koschorke, A. (2018) *Tyrants writing poetry*. Budapest: Central European Writers Press.

Kreutz, G. and Brünger, P. (2012) A shade of grey: negative associations with amateur choral singing. *Arts & Health*, 4(3), 230–38, available: https://doi.org/10.1080/17533015.2012.693111.

Lawson, B. and Phiri, M. (2003) *The architectural healthcare environment and its effect on patient outcomes*. London: London Stationary Office.

Lee, J.H. (2016) The effects of music on pain: a meta-analysis. *Journal of Music Therapy*, 53(4), 430–77.

MacDonald, R.A.R., Hargreaves, D.J. and Miell, D. (2002) *Musical identities*. Oxford: Oxford University Press.

Macklin, G. (2013) 'Onward blackshirts!': music and the British Union of Fascists. *Patterns of Prejudice*, 47(4–5), 430–57, available: https://doi.org/10.1080/0031322X.2013.845447.

Magee, W.L. (2018) Music in the diagnosis, treatment and prognosis of people with prolonged disorders of consciousness. *Neuropsychological Rehabilitation*, 28(8), 1331–9, available: https://doi.org/10.1080/09602011.2018.1494003.

Magee, W.L., Clark, I., Tamplin, J. and Bradt, J. (2017) Music interventions for acquired brain injury. *Cochrane Database of Systematic Reviews*, available: https://doi.org/10.1002/14651858.CD006787.pub3.

Magee, W.L. and O'Kelly, J. (2015) Music therapy with disorders of consciousness: current evidence and emergent evidence-based practice. *Annals of the New York Academy of Sciences*, 1337(1), 256–62, doi:10.1111/nyas.12633.

Mandoki, K. (2007) *Everyday aesthetics: prosaics, the play of culture and social identities*. London: Ashgate.

Montague, K.N., Blietz, C.M. and Kachur, M. (2009) Ensuring quieter hospital environments. *American Journal of Nursing*, 109(9), 65–7, doi: 10.1097/01.NAJ.0000360316.54373.0d.

Moss, H., Donnellan, C. and O'Neill, D. (2012) A review of qualitative methodologies used to explore patient perceptions of arts and healthcare. *Medical Humanities*, 38(2), 106–9, doi: 10.1136/medhum-2012-010196.

Moss, H., Donnellan, C. and O'Neill, D. (2015) Hospitalization and aesthetic health in older adults. *Journal of the American Medical Directors Association*, 16(2), 173.e11–173.e16, available: http://dx.doi.org/10.1016/j.jamda.2014.10.019.

Moss, H. and O'Neill, D. (2009) What training do artists need to work in healthcare settings? *Medical Humanities*, 35, 101–5, doi: 10.1136/jmh.2009.001792.

Moss, H. and O'Neill, D. (2012)Medical Humanities – Serious Academic Pursuit or Doorway to Dilettantism? *Irish Medical Journal*, 105(8), 261–2.

Moss, H. and O'Neill, D. (2014) The art of medicine: Aesthetic deprivation in clinical settings. *The Lancet*, 383(9922), 1032–3, available: https://doi.org/10.1016/S0140-6736(14)60507-9.

Moss, H. and O'Neill, D. (2016) The Role of the Curator in Modern Hospitals: A Transcontinental Perspective. *Journal of Medical Humanities*, available: https://doi. org/10.1007/s10912-016-9423-3.

O'Connell, C., Cassidy, A., O'Neill, D. and Moss, H. (2013) The Aesthetic and Cultural Pursuits of Patients with Stroke. *Journal of Stroke and Cerebrovascular Diseases*, 22(8), e404–e418, doi: 10.1016/j.jstrokecerebrovasdis.2013.04.027.

O'Neill, D., Jenkins, E., Mawhinney, R., Cosgrave, E., O'Mahony, S., Guest, C. and Moss, H. (2016) Rethinking the medical in the medical humanities. *Medical Humanities*, 42 (2), 109–14, available: http://dx.doi.org/10.1136/medhum-2015-010831.

O'Neill, D., Kelly, B., O'Keeffe, S. and Moss, H. (2020) Mainstreaming medical humanities in continuing professional development and postgraduate training. *Clinical Medicine*, 20(2), 208–211, doi: 10.7861/clinmed.2019-0332.

Ross, A. (2014) As If Music Could Do No Harm. *The New Yorker*, August 20, available: www.newyorker.com/culture/cultural-comment/music-harm.

Saito, Y. (2017) *Aesthetics of the familiar everyday life and world-making.* Oxford: Oxford University Press.

Sarkamo, T., Tervaniemi, M., Laitinen, S., Forsblom, A., Soinila, S., Mikkonen, M., Autti, T., Silvennoinen, H., Erkkila, J., Laine, M., Peretz, I. and Hietanen, M. (2008) Music listening enhances cognitive recovery and mood after middle cerebral artery stroke. *Brain*, 131, 866–76.

Shaffer, R. (2013) The soundtrack of neo-fascism: youth and music in the National Front. *Patterns of Prejudice*, 47(4–5), 458–82, available: https://doi.org/10.1080/0031322X.2013.842289.

Shapiro, J. and Rucker, L. (2003) Can poetry make better doctors? Teaching the humanities and arts to medical students and residents at the University of California, Irvine, College of Medicine. *Academic Medicine*, 78(10), 953–7.

Shekhovtsov, A. (2013) Music and the Other: an introduction. *Patterns of Prejudice*, 47(4–5), 329–35, available: http://dx.doi.org/10.1080/0031322X.2013.850801.

Sibley, F. (2001) Some notes on ugliness. In Redfern, B. and Roxbee Cox, B. eds. *Approach to aesthetics: collected papers on philosophical aesthetics*, Oxford: Clarendon Press, 2001.

Sihvonen, A.J., Särkämö, T., Leo, V., Tervaniemi, M., Altenmüller, E. and Soinila, S. (2017) Music-based interventions in neurological rehabilitation. *The Lancet Neurology*, 16(8), 648–60, available: http://dx.doi.org/10.1016/s1474-4422(17)30168-0.

Stafford Smith, C. (2008) Welcome to 'the disco'. *The Guardian*, available: www.theguardian.com/world/2008/jun/19/usa.guantanamo.

Stecker, R. (2006) Carroll's bones. *British Journal of Aesthetics*, 46, 282–6.

Stempsey, W.E. (1999) The quarantine of philosophy in medical education: why teaching the humanities may not produce humane physicians. *Medicine, Healthcare and Philosophy*, 2(1), 3–9.

Sutton, J.P. (2002) The pause that follows. *Nordic Journal of Music Therapy*, 11(1), 27–38, available: https://doi.org/10.1080/08098130209478040.

Visser, L.N.C., Tollenaar, M.S., van Doornen, L.J.P., de Haes, H.C.J.M. and Smets, E.M.A. (2019) Does silence speak louder than words? The impact of oncologists' emotion-oriented communication on analogue patients' information recall and emotional stress. *Patient Education and Counseling*, 102(1), 43–52, doi: 10.1016/j.pec.2018.08.032.

Warren, J.R. (2014) *Music and ethical responsibility*. Cambridge: Cambridge University Press.

Young, S. (2014) *I'm not your inspiration, thank you very much*. TEDtalk, available: www.ted.com/talks/stella_young_i_m_not_your_inspiration_thank_you_very_much?language=ab.

4 Excellence

Music matters in the healthcare environment

Music matters in the healthcare environment

Music has great potential to create an environment conducive to health and well-being. Dose (2006) suggests that no-one, given the choice, would actively prefer medical treatment in a setting devoid of music, or life in a community with no music provision. Research that provides compelling evidence for the arts in hospital is cited previously in this book. A wide variety of specific examples of rigorous quantitative evidence of the benefit of music in hospitals exist (to name a few, Sarkamo et al. 2008; Daykin et al. 2010; Daykin et al. 2018; Fancourt et al. 2016; Lee 2016). Several Cochrane reviews indicate evidence of the benefit of music for a variety of clinical issues presenting in hospital, albeit with the caveat that further evidence is desirable (Gold et al. 2005; Smith et al. 2006; Laopaiboon et al. 2009; Bradt and Dileo 2010a; Bradt et al. 2010b; Bradt et al. 2010c; Irons et al. 2010; Irons et al. 2019; Bradt et al. 2011; Drahota et al. 2012; Bradt et al. 2013; Jespersen et al. 2015; Magee et al. 2017; McNamara et al. 2017; van der Steen et al. 2018).

The qualitative evidence for music in healthcare is perhaps more compelling, given that such studies tend to focus on service user experience and healthcare staff acceptance of music's role in quality of care and improved well-being (MacDonald et al. 2012). The literature suggests that music in healthcare settings can contribute to a sense of wellbeing and quality of care, as well as achieve benefits in terms of service users' experience of the service. As stated in the introduction to this book, the emphasis here is to concentrate on the stress and ill health associated with aesthetically deprived environments and to normalise healthcare environments by ensuring that arts are available to service users who want them (Moss and O'Neill 2014a; Moss and O'Neill 2014b).

The arts are not about this being right or wrong. It's much more flexible than that. It is about weaving arts and creativity into the rigidness of the hospital environment and this I think softens the institution ... and it makes space for people's feelings and expression and fears, allowing them to think beyond what is happening to them.

(Kilroy et al. 2007)

Environmental aesthetics are important in making a place more of a place you want to live. It is not just about arts and music. It is about thinking about the environment in all its ways. There are things in a hospital such as communal televisions and noise pollution. What if you want to turn off the TV and someone else wants it on?

(Kirklin and Richardson 2003)

The hospital curator

The music curator has a primary role in hospital to select music that serves the function required in the hospital environment (be that to create welcome, relax people or deliver a message of care for the person).[1] However, hospitals can be conservative spaces and, in my experience, the lowest common denominator often becomes the norm, for example providing 'pleasant' 'unchallenging' art on the walls and 'light classical' music programmes. On the other hand, the curator has always held the role of introducing work that may not be well known, selecting work, offering provocation or challenge. Curators are, to a large extent, gatekeepers to the arts world (Moss and O'Neill 2019). At times I had to perform a delicate balancing act, as a curator in hospital, between promoting the intrinsic value of music and meeting both service user preferences and health service management aims for music in the environment. Challenges including persuading staff of the value of live music for their service users and finding space where 'noisy' drums could be played. The growth of online music streaming has also created a new function for the music curator, who no longer provides music to listen to (for we can access whatever we want online) but must select which music to bring to public attention. My research of the aesthetic enrichment in the hospital evidenced that most service users had no control over whether the TV or radio was on in their ward or room, nor which channel they would watch and were faced with noise pollution daily and no access to any of their normal aesthetic interest. At best their aesthetic needs were neglected, at worst they were aesthetically deprived.

The debate about the value of music in healthcare settings can be seen as a split between politicians and policy makers who value the 'instrumental value' of the arts and cultural professionals who are dedicated to the 'intrinsic value' of the particular medium. This debate has been seen throughout the history of aesthetics (Gaut and McIver Lopes 2005; Kieran 2005). The debate can also be seen in the curatorial aspects of arts in healthcare settings. Are the arts provided to meet certain health promotion or clinical aims or are they intrinsically valuable in healthcare contexts?

Curators inside healthcare contexts have a delicate role in balancing support for the intrinsic value of the arts with meeting service users' preferences and health service aims for improved well-being through the arts. Clearly articulated aims are paramount in this emerging field. I have identified twelve considerations for successful music curation in hospital which will be discussed here.

1. Musical choice and control

Healthcare settings are one of few environments in modern society that can be devoid of the arts. There is little expectation that one can continue their arts (and indeed any leisure) activities in health settings when they are ill. It is the contention of this book that rather than needing evidence to prove the benefit of the arts for health and well-being, we need simply to attest to the effect of aesthetic neglect on well-being in healthcare institutions. The process of hospitalisation is known to commonly create feelings of fear, doubt, helplessness, loss of control, and increases in stress and anxiety (Barnason et al. 1995). Increased anxiety has negative physiological effects on the heart, including elevated cortisol and adrenaline, which correspond with increased heart rate and blood pressure (Selle and Silverman 2017). Choice and control over music choices (for service users and staff) can alleviate feelings of helplessness and fear.

Loss of choice and control is experienced at many levels in hospital. For example, you may have no choice about whether a TV is on or off in the ward or what time breakfast is served, no option to make tea or coffee when you want, no control over the events and appointments of the day or what time a doctor will visit. There is a loss of feeling safe and secure (are my valuables safe in the bedside locker? Will a confused service user invade my personal space? Is my body going to survive this crisis?). Then there are even more minor, subtle losses, such as lack of choice of bed linen (replaced by institutional hospital sheets); loss of my own favourite mug to have coffee in the morning (replaced by one of one hundred identical, cheap white mugs which are used in hospitals), lack of choice over the time of day I go to sleep and wake up, lack of choice over which radio station is blaring on the ward (Mandoki 2007; Saito 2008; Moss et al. 2015).

Caspari (2018) has explored the deprivation and loss of dignity that occurs when nursing home residents are denied choice and freedom over their daily activities. 'When one is denied the opportunity to participate or is "forced" to participate in activities that one does not enjoy, dignity is essentially threatened' (Slettebø et al. 2017; Caspari et al. 2018). It is known that although being in a single room or a multiple bed ward does not make a significant difference to the recovery rate of service users, those clients who are in the type of accommodation of their <u>own choice</u> feel more satisfied with their treatment and make better progress than those who are not (Lawson 2001).

Studies of the negative effect of the arts in healthcare settings are few. However, there has been increasing concern over the use of music in the operating room as a distraction to staff. In one study, it was found that music may contribute to overall level of background noise and impair effective communication among members of the surgical team (Cruise et al. 1997). Music choices can offer a simple but effective way to validate individuality and offer freedom in a hospital environment.

Peter's story

I met Peter in a forensic mental health setting, where he was hospitalised following a trial for murder. He was found not guilty by reason of insanity and had a diagnosis of paranoid schizophrenia. Coupled with a drink and drug binge weekend, his paranoid thoughts had resulted in the horrific murder of his mother. He was only twenty years old. Peter's life in the secure unit was tightly controlled, the aim of his treatment was to gain insight into his offence and his mental health issues. Peter attended individual music therapy with me for a year. He loved to play the drums, loudly and boisterously and treated the music therapy room rather like a room full of toys. There was something very youthful about Peter, he rarely sat still, had little concentration and was full of energy.

The music therapy sessions involved improvisation and talking. During improvisations I attempted to connect with him in the music and to discuss afterwards how the music felt, encouraging reflectiveness and honesty in his conversations. Music therapy often acted as a precursor to verbal therapy, especially with service users who found talking therapy extremely difficult. Music therapy offered an enjoyable forum in which to build a trusting relationship with a therapist.

The key aspect of this therapy however, for Peter and for the majority of clients in a forensic setting, was the choice offered to them in the music therapy room. All other aspects of their lives were locked down, structured and pre-determined. Their freedom was literally restricted, physically and psychologically. Music therapy offered a window in the week when choices could be made and explorations of self-control could be made safely (how hard can I hit this drum safely without losing control?). Music affords a freedom of expression and choice-making opportunity in the most controlled of atmospheres.

2. Musical safety and security

Lawson's (2001) seminal work on the psychology of space identified three psychological needs we all have in any space – to be secure, to be stimulated and to have a sense of one's own identity. A sense of safety and identity can be reinforced in hospital through musical choices and expression. Music therapists work with people with dementia, for example, to select songs based on previous experiences and preferences, to offer safety, familiarity and personal significance in a time of confusion. The skilful work of a music professional in hospital is in creating a safe space in which musical activity can take place whilst also stimulating new ideas and discoveries when appropriate. This delicate dance must take account of the power of music to transcend normal life, affect our mood, cause division and challenge us. We want to know that this musical vulnerability is not going to be exploited (Levitin 2008). Teaching parents to sing lullabies with their hospitalised babies was one of the simplest and yet most profound experiences of my practice.

3. Musical stimulation

Hospitals usually aim to offer security and a sense of safety and reassurance rather than stimulation, but for long-term service users stimulation is also important. Lawson (2003) states that hospital spaces need to do what they seldom do; they need to counteract the loss of independence and identity the service user feels. 'A common mistake is to concentrate too much on the central purpose of the space and thus to forget the rest of the human condition. Such a way of thinking leads to the wonderfully efficient and clinically sterile hospital that treats the body and yet numbs the spirit' (Lawson 2003).

Music offers a wonderfully accessible source of stimulation, for example, encouraging physical exercise (how many of us exercise to music in the gym?), cognitive stimulation (song lyric recall) and socialising.

4. Musical identity

The fear of losing one's identity and becoming 'a number on a chart' was a persistent feature of my work with service users in hospital (Moss and O'Neill 2014). Tapping into personal preferences and meaningful leisure activities is an important part of clinical care. A life review through music (creating a playlist of memorable music moments throughout the person's life) is a simple but effective way to counter this fear of invisibility. As explored thoroughly in *Musical Identities*, music plays an important role in the everyday lives of ordinary people – as consumers, fans, listeners, composers, arrangers, performers, and critics (MacDonald et al. 2002). Music is used not only as a means by which people formulate and express their individual identities and present themselves to others, but also by individuals to regulate their own everyday moods and behaviours.

In 2007, I conducted one of my first pieces of research to evaluate the benefit of live music in hospital in collaboration with the Irish Chamber Orchestra (Moss et al. 2007). The study hoped to shed some light on which music was preferable within an acute hospital context and there was a desire from healthcare staff to find the 'best' relaxing music. When 1,000 stakeholders were surveyed, we discovered that every single genre of music was listed as 'relaxing'. Suggestions ranged from Eminem to heavy metal to 'middle of the road classical' to country and western music. This study confirms extensive research indicating that defining 'relaxing' music is futile. Personally preferred music is recommended for people recovering from illness (Mitchell and MacDonald 2006; Garza-Villarreal et al. 2014; Fidler and Miksza 2020). I have yet to meet an individual who cannot name their favourite music or music with personal meaning, nor have I ever met two people with exactly the same musical tastes. Retaining a sense of one's individuality and identity is reported by many writers to be important in their illness and recovery journey (Bauby 2004; Carel 2016; Gleeson 2019; Robins 2019).

5. Compassionate care

Music offers a simple and effective way to offer compassion and individual care in healthcare institutions. Two examples follow.

Claire's story

Claire is a 25- year-old woman I met in an acute psychiatry unit. Working with the Occupational Therapist, I established a music therapy service, offering a singing group at 10 a.m. every Monday morning on the ward for anyone who had been admitted over the weekend (commonly emergency admissions such as suicide risk, self harm or psychotic episodes). My aim for this group was to offer a non-threatening space that people could use for 5 minutes or 50, depending on their need and ability to tolerate being with other people, concentrate and engage. The group acted as part of the assessment of the new resident's needs and difficulties and fed into a wider team assessment process. Having offered more in-depth group processes to service users, this group grew from an awareness that many people on the ward found group work challenging and were wary of engaging in groups with esoteric titles such as 'music therapy' or 'improvisation' and might feel incompetent when facing a 'song writing' or 'choir' group. Hence this group was simply an opportunity to sing or listen to others singing.

The format of the group was designed to be as accessible as possible. I started by playing some soft music on piano while we waited for people to join us and made light conversation with people who arrived, saying hello, asking their name and what sort of music they enjoyed listening to. When the group began, I would begin some of the following activities:

- Welcome everyone to the group
- Set the boundaries of the group (most importantly, what time the group ended and that it was okay to come and go if people needed to and to participate only if they felt comfortable and wanted to)
- Pass a drum and introduce yourself to the group
- Ask people if there was a song they particularly liked. Engage in conversation and either sing the song as a group or ask them to share a little of the song
- Open with some familiar well-known songs that I either sang to the group (if no one wanted to sing) or led the group who would join in
- Ask people to think of the first song they remember as a child and who sang it to them. Where this was a positive memory, we would recreate this song by singing it together. Careful curation of this activity was necessary as some people may never have had this experience or may have forgotten it
- Mindful meditation using music – I would play piano using two repetitive chords, slow and soft and give directions to breathe and relax. Most often, I used this at the end of the session if the atmosphere felt chaotic, to try and ensure that people returned to the ward calm and/or if people were highly anxious
- Chime bar exercise – each patient had a chime bar and again I would play soft repetitive grounding chords and rhythm, and people were invited to join in if they wanted and play the chime bar. Chime bars make a lovely sound but cannot really override other people so allow equality (where someone has been overly dominant) and can create a calm overall effect. White notes were used so that clashes were minimal

The group ranged from being a predominantly receptive experience (whereby people listened to songs being sung by me) to highly interactive and led by group members, where the group would sing, chat and bond over shared singing and musical interests. Group membership ranged from one person attending to eight. Instruments were available and if appropriate I would invite people to play instruments while singing and improvise but the emphasis was on no pressure.

Claire had a diagnosis of post-natal psychosis[2] (Health Service Executive 2019). She attended the group and happened to be the only person this Monday morning. She appeared very withdrawn, looked tired and sad. When asked how she was she said she was really missing her children. I asked their ages – they were aged twenty-two months and one month old. She offered that her partner has been amazing; she wished he knew how amazing he was and how much she loved him. I didn't know if others would join us – the first 15 minutes allowed for drop-in so I began by playing some songs that Claire liked and invited her to relax and listen as well. She didn't sing herself but said the music was lovely. It became apparent that no-one else was joining the group. At this point, I decided to take the opportunity to offer Claire support as she had raised some poignant issues. She did not want to sing herself, so I asked her if she might like to write a song for her partner. She said she would like to thank him for his support. I chose a basic chord progression (too many questions at this stage would have been diffi-cult for her cognitively and emotionally as she was extremely low in mood). I simply began to play some repetitive chords and asked her to tell me a few things about her partner. She offered that he was kind, caring and stood by her side. He was a fantastic father and he was looking after her girls. She said she wanted to thank him and tell him she would be home soon. I sang these words, improvising a song for her. I ensured that I reflected back her words and sentiments, did not overly interpret just gave them a musical expression. The result was a beautiful song to her partner and she loved it. She cried but smiled through the tears.

We had only one session, which was a pity, as this session showed much potential for Claire to use music to explore her feelings and express herself. However, I believe this session was a moment of hope for Claire in the midst of a very dark time in her life.

It is important to reiterate here that music can have a negative effect and cause distress (See Chapter 3). A skilled, registered music therapist using music in appropriate ways within healthcare contexts with vulnerable people can select and facilitate music safely.

Nora's story

I met Nora in a ward for older people with medical and mental health issues in Berkshire, England in the late 1990s. Nora had advanced dementia and was an in-patient having had a bad fall. She was referred to music therapy as she was isolated, did not receive many visitors and was extremely quiet and withdrawn.

The Occupational Therapist carried out an assessment of all new service users, including an interview with their next of kin. Part of her assessment included listing their musical preferences. Nora did not have a list, as she had no next of kin and was not able to recall and explain her preferences during the assessment. I met Nora in the music therapy room and during her assessment session I played a few well-known pieces of music, from different genres, to see if I could make a connection. I noticed as I wheeled her to the room that she said she sang in the church choir. Over the first two weeks of sessions I realised this was the only information I was receiving about her. In my desperation I asked her the name of the church. A stroke of luck – the church she named was familiar to me and I knew it to be Roman Catholic. So, I plucked the one Catholic hymn I knew, *The Bells of the Angelus*, and played the opening bars. Nora sat up, started singing and never stopped! From then on, we shared hymns that she knew and talked a little about her memories of the church choir.

Following this break-through session, I spoke to the nurse in charge on the ward. No connection had been made with the Catholic chaplain in the hospital as Nora had not been identified as Roman Catholic on admission. A referral was made to the pastoral care department and Nora began to receive regular visits from the Catholic community.

I have never forgotten this brief, but intense, relationship with Nora. It taught me a fundamental lesson – if we can connect with someone through music, we can illuminate the person's true identity. Everyone has musical preferences. It is rare to find someone without a musical memory, or a significant song. Many can compile a *life review* using music (Sato 2011).

Several studies report the need for clinical staff to treat service users as individuals in order to enhance their experience of care. Grover et al. (2018) for example interviewed people with cancer in hospital. They wanted staff to approach them as individuals first and then as persons with cancer, to be considerate of their roles (socially and occupationally) beyond the 'sick' role. Bramley and Matiti (2014) define compassionate care as 'knowing me and giving me your time, knowing what it is like in my shoes and communicating with me'. But why does this matter? Some would argue that being kind, giving time to service users, makes no difference to recovery rate, pain medication used or effectiveness of surgery or treatment and that funding would better be spent on treating a person efficiently than giving them 20 minutes to tell their story and cry in the clinic. These contradictory positions are extreme. However, my experience attests to the benefit of the arts in helping people feel comfortable and cared for, valued and individual in healthcare spaces and research indicates benefits in reducing recovery time and levels of pain medication (Ulrich 1992; Devlin and Arneill 2003; Ulrich and Gilpin 2003; Jonas and Chez 2004; Codinhoto et al. 2009; Huisman et al. 2012). More research is needed in this area.

6. Music to make meaning out of serious illness

Major illnesses require rehabilitation, recovery and adaptation to a new reality. One service user described this journey as an adjustment to a totally new way of being and doing:

> Adjustment to disability involves understanding, exploring, responding and working through a range of loss and grief and forming a new identity.
>
> (Baker and Wigram 2005)

When people can tell a story to reflect and express their experiences, and when these are heard and acknowledged by others, there is hope for improved coping and making sense of illness. Music can be a useful story-telling tool, with the function of emotional processing, social integration of experiences, and re-establishing an organised whole. There are many studies that underpin the power of storytelling as a way of 'meaning making' not only for ill people (Bury 1982; Bolton 1999; Bury 2001; Charon 2001; Bolton 2005; Charon 2006; Charon 2013; Carel 2016; Carel 2018). Morris (2008) presents the idea of rebuilding identity from the lens of a community-based rehabilitation therapist, noting the limitations of defining such an illness or event as 'incurable', and examining the need to reconfigure one's identity post-injury or traumatic event. Like any other loss experience, there are phases of grief and a new view of what 'healthy' means, leading to a state of enhanced well-being, albeit with an altered story of one's identity.

> Hope does not mean a cure; hope can simply mean hope for a better day
>
> (Robins 2019)

7. Musical self-reflection

Music, and indeed all the arts, enable us to explore the deeper mysteries of the human condition, which may explain the high value placed on arts by all societies. Certainly, the role of music as part of medical and health human-ities, to draw out experiences and reflect on them, is well explored.

> The arts must be taken no less seriously than the sciences as modes of discovery, creation and enlargement of knowledge in the broad sense of advancement of the understanding.
>
> (Graham 1997)

Two recent examples of the role of music to enable reflection and understanding follow. Paul Noonan's original song reflects on the experience of dementia, with a beautiful film created by Lochlainn McKenna.

> Listen and watch online 4.1: Glacier by Paul Noonan, video directed by Lochlainn McKenna www.youtube.com/watch?v=efOc__m9Jy8

'Maura', by Daniel Dineen, is a song created for a student project as part of his MA Music Therapy qualification, to reflect on the experience of a client Maura, who has high levels of anxiety and is socially isolated. Maura is 66 years old and lives alone in a small one-bedroom flat in a town centre, attends a day centre but refuses to participate in any group programmes. She likes country and western music. Her anxiety disorder impacts all areas of her life. This song was created to reflect on life from Maura's point of view as part of a student assignment to encourage and enable greater understanding of the perspective of the service user.

> Listen and watch online 4.2: Maura by Daniel Dineen* see list of online files for access details on p. ix.

8. Music as pleasure and respite from the difficulties of everyday hospital life

Hume (1711–1776) is one of the foremost philosophers to hold the view that music (and the arts) are primarily connected with pleasure or enjoyment (Graham 1997). Schopenhauer (1778–1860) identified the ability of music (and the arts) to provide escapism or respite from the trials of everyday life. Music plays a pivotal role in life by allowing us a temporary respite from the cares of daily life; a transcendence of practical desire and a breaking free from the servitude of the will and the suffering of life (Graham 1997). In healthcare scenarios, I used music many times to lift the atmosphere on a ward, to bring people a moment of respite from the bleak acute hospital ward experience. The music alone can lift a person to a new, better place, even for a moment and this instillation of hope, or simply distraction, can be crucial in coping with difficult moments in our lives.

An over emphasis on music as merely amusement or recreation might explain why musicians often struggle to have a serious role in healthcare settings, and why music therapists often fight the perception that they provide just 'a good sing song'. Issues such as low funding available in healthcare to pay highly qualified professional musicians stems from this perspective on music. Nonetheless, it is important to acknowledge that people rarely expect to have fun while in hospital and this can be highly positive. In a bleak time of life, it is possible to have a fleeting moment of fun.

9. Music as emotional expression

The emotional and communicative aspects of music are significant.

> Art is a human activity consisting in this, that one man consciously by means of certain external signs, hands on to others feelings he has lived through, and that others are affected by these feelings and also experience them.
>
> (Tolstoy 1930, p. 106)

The ability of artists, musicians and poets to arouse dangerous emotions was one of the factors that led Plato to ban them from his ideal Republic. It is possible that one can never really separate the aesthetic experience from personal experience and emotion, for example a song heard at a funeral of someone we love takes on a totally different role in our lives and is appreciated in a different way to the same song heard prior to this event. Music therapy deals substantially with the emotional aspects of music. The ability of music to affect mood, release tears, express frustration and anger is a powerful tool in accessing the person's experience. Song writing, for example, is a particularly powerful form of storytelling for people with limited verbal communication and serious illness.

10. Music as beauty and hope

Music can offer a moment of beauty, hope and transcendence where experience is dark and difficult. Even in the most abused, damaged individuals I have worked with, I have seen a tiny spark of creativity in the artwork they produce or the music they play. This offers a critical moment of hope and shows a potential. I firmly believe that in every individual there is creativity, hope and a future. The role of the arts in creating moments of hope and beauty and transforming negative experiences through the arts is important and often neglected in healthcare settings. Notarangelo (2019) argues that the human propensity to use music for transcendent purposes exists whether or not it is given overt clinical focus by music therapists.

The concept of beauty appears to have little attention or importance in modern society, and it is rarely mentioned in hospital planning. 'It is tempting to drop the talk about beauty altogether, and steer the discussion toward more quantifiable matters: cost, sustainability, economic benefits, and so forth' (Parsons 2010). Beauty is about transcending the everyday and finding meaning and our spiritual core. In terms of curating music in hospital, it is important to bear witness to the possibility that live music can transport the listener somewhere beautiful, above the everyday mess to a moment of reprieve and release. At one live performance at the hospital a man with a stroke said to me 'I've been to physiotherapy, to see the doctor, the nurse, the occupational therapist. They are all brilliant and they are curing me. But this … this music … this is the cure for the soul' (Moss et al. 2007).

Whether beauty matters, and what beauty is, are subjective concepts and in healthcare settings beauty can be an afterthought, an item on an agenda that prioritises efficiency, cost reduction and safety. Accounts by people with illness tell a different story. A glimpse of hope and beauty, perhaps through live music, is needed psychologically as a reminder that it exists, despite the imperfections of the world and the difficulties being experienced at the time. Transcendence is a word that has frequently been ascribed to music, lifting us from our misery and offering hope. 'To live with beauty is to live in the world we want, a world where, despite the obstacles, at least some good thing has flourished beyond our imagination. It is not difficult to see the deep psychological satisfaction that this kind of experience can offer' (Parsons 2010).

11. Music as an interdisciplinary activity

Collaboration with clinical staff was crucial to my success as a hospital curator. I am sure that no project I undertook and delivered happened alone, and the very best projects grew from collaborations. Doctors are more likely than the average person to learn a musical instrument or be a painter (O'Neill et al. 2016), and although I had been assigned the role of 'the arts person' in hospital I soon realised that the hospital was filled with artists, musicians, actors and so on, amongst all staff groups and service users. Artists bring their skills just as nurses, doctors and service users bring their expertise to the table. The best arts projects were a collaboration between all these stakeholders (Fitzgerald and Callard 2015). Two examples follow.

Mindful Music

Mindful music was an initiative developed with staff and students at a university teaching hospital. A lunchtime slot was advertised, and people were invited to drop in, informally, to de-stress, unwind and relax using music and mindfulness. Mindfulness exercises and live music were combined to provide a simple, accessible self-care session for staff. Music students from the academy on campus joined us to co-facilitate the session. We ended each session with a song (usually Let it Be by the Beatles) to encourage a lift of energy before people returned to work and to allow for communal singing which we believed could enhance feelings of wellness, positivity and relaxation. The session has been provided in online format also and is being researched to document its positive outcomes.

Niamh's story

Dr Niamh Bohane is a GP and a writer. She bravely shares here her experience of the power of music to support her in a difficult health moment. Her experience sums up many of the themes above, namely the importance of music as a means of self-expression, respite, beauty and hope and the importance of understanding that clinical staff have responses to the arts and expertise in this area also.

Since I was a child, music has been my comfort and words my business. It was music that soothed me through the internal turbulence of growing up but it was stories that allowed me to communicate with the outside world. I sang and played piano in private, soul swimming in the notes and intervals. I wrote stories and articles, my brain sharing ideas and thoughts about the world. So when, several years ago, I reached a state of burnout in my job as a doctor, I tried to write my way through, trusting that my brain would lead me out of this. I sat with journals and advisers; I asked myself questions and tried to answer those of others. But with all my efforts, the words wouldn't come. When I really needed them, they failed me. Putting words to the feelings I had seemed like a betrayal of the career I'd worked for, the people I served, the family who supported me. I just could not speak or write what I felt. A friend who knew my hidden musical love suggested I play it out. "What a lovely idea but I have a serious problem here," I joked, but only because it was easier that admitting I was scared. I had only ever sung or played other people's music. Where would I even start? Not long after, my throat and chest choked up with anxiety and stress and my words almost completely silenced, I crawled back to her. "How would I do that?"

She gave me a recording of a guided singing technique to try. One desperate day, I listened and, cheeks burning even in the silence on my own, I tried. First one interval, then the next, adding a few together, moving up and down scales, repeating patterns that felt soothing and cathartic. Once I started, it was hard to stop. Emotions so desperately needing a valve found an escape. Tears and notes flowed together.

It was as if I'd found a new language that allowed me to express the things I needed to say without hurting or blaming anything or anyone, including myself. Finally, when the dam of sadness had been burst, I was able to see my problems, now washed clean of overwhelming emotions, for what they were, put names to them, acknowledge them and start to address them. Words served me again but only because music had ministered to me in the valley of tears.

12. Musical community

Social singing demonstrates the role of music in reducing isolation and benefits are well documented (Clift et al. 2008; Clift and Hancox 2010; Clift, Hancox, et al. 2010; Clift, Nichol, et al. 2010; Irons et al. 2010; Fancourt and Perkins 2017; Goldenberg 2017; Moss et al. 2017a; Moss et al. 2017b; Bonde et al. 2018; Daykin et al. 2018; Dingle et al. 2019). The hospital workplace choir I established saw over fifty members of staff join and it is flourishing today. At the weekly choir rehearsal after work, doctors stood next to porters, cleaners next to nurse managers, healthcare assistants next to Speech and Language therapists. The choir is a place to relax, sing your heart out, laugh, meet new people at work, build community and achieve performances that you never dreamed were possible (Moss et al. 2017a; Moss and O'Donoghue 2018).

Chronic illness can be a lonely experience. Many of the hospital service user groups I worked with found most benefit from the social and peer support found in arts groups (O'Neill and Moss 2015; Fitzpatrick et al. 2019). Hospital can be a lonely place, where one is part of a community of circumstance rather than a community of participation (Ansdell 2014). The Monday morning group (described earlier in this chapter) allowed service users in an acute psychiatry ward to begin to form a tentative community. Sometimes it is easier to be part of a musical group than a verbal one, especially when words and eye contact are difficult (Pavlicevic 2003).

Examples of excellence: aesthetic enrichment through music

Three examples are signposted here, recognised nationally and internationally as examples of good practice. No recommendations can be comprehensive and excellent examples will surely have been omitted. However, these three music health services are chosen as they inspired this author to strive for creativity and excellence. The hope is that these examples will stimulate discussion and enthuse readers to find many other good examples which undoubtedly exist.

The Louis Armstrong Center for Music and Medicine at Mount Sinai Beth Israel, New York City.

The world-renowned MT department at the Mount Sinai Health System has multiple programmes including in-patient music therapy with both service users and their families; numerous research projects co-investigated with doctors and nurses, an extensive outpatient MT clinic and a service for musicians, performing artists and others prone to depression, overuse, focal dystonia and performance anxiety. The department has a strong clinical training component and their faculty lecture globally and have assisted in the expansion of music therapy in hospitals and clinics across the globe. Their research has been featured in medical and music therapy journals and in the media. Led by Prof Joanne Loewy, the centre hosts musicians in their Visiting Artists Program where musicians are trained to provide music in the lobbies of the hospitals.

> Listen and watch online 4.3: The Louis Armstrong Department of Music Therapy, Mount Sinai Beth Israel, New York City www.mountsinai.org/locations/music-therapy

The Chelsea and Westminster Hospital NHS Foundation Trust (CWNHS)

This hospital delivers both an MT service and music programme which co-exist and are funded separately. The renowned music therapy service at the hospital provides music therapy to children who need support to develop their communication, social interaction, emotional and motor skills, enabling the creative expression of feelings and ability to engage in shared musical play with others. Integrated packages of outpatient individual and group music therapy are offered to children as part of a multi-disciplinary Child Development Service (Wood et al. 2016; Flower and Watts 2019). This leading music therapy service is jointly led by Juliet Wood and Claire Flower. The team have also initiated a unique environmental music therapy service in the maternity ward (Flower and Watts 2018; Flower and Meadows 2019). Overall this music therapy service is an example of effective and thoughtful development of specialised musical activities and interventions, in collaboration with service users and multi-disciplinary team, using music and music therapy to improve the experience of care received by service users and their families.

> Listen and watch online 4.4: Music Therapy at the Chelsea and Westminster Hospital NHS Foundation Trust www.chelwest.nhs.uk/services/therapy-services/childrens-therapy/music-therapy.

The hospital charity CW+ manages a comprehensive arts programme, including several leading examples of music in hospital. Programmes include a hospital music app to accompany the hospital's visual art tour (15 composers were commissioned); a sophisticated personal listening system, installed in almost every waiting and treatment room, which offers seven playlist choices, themed as classical, jazz, golden oldies, paediatric, ambient, guitar and piano (service users can control the volume, whether the music is on or off and what sort of music they wish to listen to). CW+ also invests in several musicians in residence, including a hospital pianist, violinist and harpist and has commissioned several new 'soundscapes' for the Imaging Department. These soundscapes are created for each waiting area in order to give each one a distinct sonic identity, making them easily identifiable. CW+ has also developed a mobile app called OPRA (the Older People's Rhythm App) which affords service users who must remain in bed to engage in group music-making workshops that they cannot physically attend (Scott et al. 2019).

Listen and watch online 4.5: CW+ Art and Design programme www. cwplus.org.uk/our-work/art-and-design/ and https://www.cwplus. org.uk.

National Centre for Arts and Health, Tallaght University Hospital, Dublin (NCAH)

This music programme is part of a renowned arts and health programme led by Alison Baker, Arts Manager/Curator (NCAH). Senior Music Therapist and Music Co-ordinator Clara Monahan co-ordinates a wide variety of musical experiences for all ages across many clinical departments, as well as providing a music therapy service in the older age wards (Baker 2019). The programme has evolved to include live performance, music therapy, musicians in residence and composers, all working alongside each other in complementary ways. Professional and volunteer musicians co-exist and all musicians are vetted, trained and approved before performing and attend ongoing training and support throughout their time at the hospital. Programmes range from performances, where musicians have minimal contact with service users and play 'in the background' of clinical areas, to music therapy in psychiatry, older age and paediatric wards, which is based on clinical referral and delivered as part of the multi-disciplinary team. An award winning hospital workplace choir is well established, as well as the 'Sing while you can Singers', a casual singing group developed in conjunction with Pastoral Care staff to offer support and care to staff and service users. A musician in residence project called 'Soothing Sounds' for parents

and children in the paediatric service adds another dimension to the programme and the hospital was the first in Ireland to host an orchestra and
composer in residence.

> Listen and watch online 4.6: National Centre for Arts and
> Health, Tallaght University Hospital, Dublin four-year review
> 2016–2020 and Arts Department, National Centre for Arts and
> Health, Tallaght University Hospital, Dublin www.youtube.com/
> watch?v=1n8laWfAmuQ; and https://www.tuh.ie/Departments/
> Arts-Department-%E2%80%93-National-Centre-for-Arts-and-
> Health and www.tuh.ie/!ZZMFR4.

Final thoughts

This chapter set out the areas that need to be considered when curating
music in hospitals and signposted three world class examples. Deci and
Ryan's Self-Determination Theory (2012) is a useful reference point in
bringing this chapter to a conclusion. They define the psychological needs
of humans as relatedness (the need to connect socially and be integrated in
a social group); competence (the need to be effective in one's efforts) and
autonomy (one needs to feel one's activities are self-governed, self-endorsed
and of free will). Securing these needs will go far in enabling a sense of a
person's own identity and power (Deci and Ryan 2012; Welch et al. 2019).
Tom's experience was the antithesis of this vision.

Tom's story

Tom was a traditional Irish dancer in his leisure time, with a huge passion
for dance and active in his local community supporting young people to
develop a love of dance. At the age of 64 Tom had a stroke that left him with
brain injury and impaired hearing and in need of disability support services.
He retired from his work in insurance. He summed up his experience of the
health service and the related loss of his identity and opportunity to dance:

> I am a client of the health service – but I would like my professionals to
> acknowledge my vast experience. I am also a dancer. I hear very little
> about this.
>   Yes, we are there to be served but we have life experience and it's
> humiliating when we are not seen, when our skills are not acknowledged,
> when we are not known.
>   Everyone has the right to dance but many people are denied that.
> Older people are not encouraged to dance. They are encouraged to sit

still and behave. I want to be alive and I want to be free. I can't wait and I'm not going to wait, for regulation, for health and safety assessments, to be put in a box. I cannot wait and I dare not wait. Inside I'm dancing and I'll scream if you say we are thinking about this, we'll look into it, we'll work on it.

The next chapter explores the professional issues to consider in the field.

Notes

1 The word 'curator' comes from the Latin word *curare*, meaning to take care. In Roman times, it meant to take care of the bath houses, in medieval times, it designated the priest who cared for souls. Later, in the eighteenth century, it meant looking after collections of art and artifacts. Modern curating, including music curation, involves displaying and facilitating access to arts, and enabling mass engagement through internet, live interaction and recordings (Jeffries and Groves 2014).

2 Postpartum psychosis is a rare and severe form of postnatal depression. It is also called postnatal or puerperal psychosis. Postpartum psychosis happens within the first few weeks after giving birth, and can begin as early as 2 to 3 days after childbirth. Symptoms of postpartum psychosis include feeling paranoid, having delusions or hallucinations, mood swings and confused thinking and associated changes in behaviour. You are most at risk of developing postpartum psychosis if you have an existing mental health condition.

References

Ansdell, G. (2014) *How music helps in music therapy and everyday life*. Farnham: Ashgate.

Baker, A. (2019) *National Centre for Arts and Health: Arts and Health Programme Four Year Review*, Tallaght University Hospital, Dublin, Ireland: Tallaght University Hospital, available: www.artsandhealth.ie/wp-content/uploads/2019/12/Tallaght-University-Hospital-Four-Year-Arts-Review-2015-2018.pdf.

Baker F. and Wigram T. eds. (2005) *Songwriting: methods, techniques and clinical applications for music therapy clinicians, educators and students*. London: Jessica Kingsley.

Barnason, S., Zimmerman, L. and Nieveen, J. (1995) The effects of music interventions on anxiety in the patient after coronary artery bypass grafting. *Heart Lung*, 24(2), 124–32, available: http://dx.doi.org/10.1016/s0147-9563(05)80007-x.

Bauby, J.-D. (2004) *The diving-bell and the butterfly*. London: Harper Perennial.

Bolton, G. (1999) *Therapeutic potential of creative writing*. London: Jessica Kingsley.

Bolton, G. (2005) *Reflective practice: writing and professional development*, 2nd ed., London: Sage.

Bonde, L.O., Juel, K. and Ekholm, O. (2018) Associations between music and health-related outcomes in adult non-musicians, amateur musicians and professional musicians—Results from a nationwide Danish study. *Nordic Journal of Music*

Therapy, 27(4), 262–82, available: www.tandfonline.com/doi/abs/10.1080/08098131.2018.1439086.

Bradt, J. and Dileo, C. (2010a) Music therapy for end-of-life care. *Cochrane Database of Systematic Reviews*.

Bradt, J., Dileo, C. and Grocke, D. (2010b) Music interventions for mechanically ventilated patients. *Cochrane Database of Systematic Reviews*.

Bradt, J., Dileo, C., Grocke, D. and Magill, L. (2011) Music interventions for improving psychological and physical outcomes in cancer patients (review). *Cochrane Database of Systematic Reviews*.

Bradt, J., Dileo, C. and Potvin, N. (2013) Music for stress and anxiety reduction in coronary heart disease patients. *Cochrane Database of Systematic Reviews*, available: http://dx.doi.org/10.1002/14651858.CD006577.pub3.

Bradt, J., Magee W.L., Dileo, C., Wheeler, L. and McGilloway, E. (2010c) Music therapy for acquired brain injury. *Cochrane Database of Systematic Reviews*.

Bramley, L. and Matiti, M. (2014) How does it really feel to be in my shoes? Patients' experiences of compassion within nursing care and their perceptions of developing compassionate nurses. *Journal of Clinical Nursing*, 23(19–20), 2790–99, available: https://doi.org/10.1111/jocn.12537.

Bury, M. (1982) Chronic illness as biographical disruption. *Sociology of Health and Illness*, 4, 167–82.

Bury, M. (2001) Illness narratives: fact or fiction? *Sociology of Health & Illness*, 23(3), 263–85, available: https://doi.org/10.1111/1467-9566.00252.

Carel, H. (2016) *Phenomenology of illness*. Oxford: Oxford University Press.

Carel, H. (2018) *Illness: the cry of the flesh*, 3rd ed. Abingdon: Routledge.

Caspari, S., Råholm, M.B., Sæteren, B., Rehnsfeldt, A., Lillestø, B., Lohne, V., Slettebø, Å., Heggestad, A.K.T., Høy, B., Lindwall, L. and Nåden, D. (2018) Tension between freedom and dependence—A challenge for residents who live in nursing homes. *Journal of Clinical Nursing*, 27(21–22), 4119–27, available: http://dx.doi.org/10.1111/jocn.14561.

Charon, R. (2001) Narrative Medicine: A Model for Empathy, Reflection, Profession, and Trust. *JAMA: The Journal of the American Medical Association*, 286(15), 1897–902, doi:10.1001/jama.286.15.1897.

Charon, R. (2006) *Narrative medicine: honoring the stories of illness*. New York: Oxford University Press.

Charon, R. (2013) Narrative medicine in the international education of physicians. *La Presse Médicale*, 42(1), 3–5.

Clift, S. and Hancox, G. (2010) The significance of choral singing for sustaining psychological wellbeing: findings from a survey of choristers in England, Australia and Germany. *Music Performance Research*, 3(1), 79–96.

Clift, S., Hancox, G., Morrison, I., Hess, B., Kreutz, G. and Stewart, D. (2010) Choral singing and psychological wellbeing: Quantitative and qualitative findings from English choirs in a cross-national survey. *Journal of Applied Arts & Health*, 1(1), 19–34, available: https://doi.org/10.1386/jaah.1.1.19/1.

Clift, S., Hancox, G., Staricoff, R., Whitmore, C., Morrison, I. and Raisbeck, M. (2008) *Singing and health: summary of a systematic mapping and review of non-clinical research.* Canterbury: Canterbury Christ Church University, available: www.canterbury.ac.uk/centres/sidney-de-haan-research/.

Clift, S., Nicol, J., Raisbeck, M., Whitmore, C. and Morrison, I. (2010) Group singing, wellbeing and health: a systematic mapping of research evidence. *Multi-Disciplinary Research in the Arts*, 2(1), 1–25.

Codinhoto, R., Tzortzopoulos, P., Kagioglou, M., Aouad, G. and Cooper, R. (2009) The impacts of the built environment on health outcomes. *Facilities*, 27(3/4), 138–51, available: http://dx.doi.org/10.1108/02632770910933152.

Cruise, C.J., Chung, F., Yogendran, S. and Little, D.A. (1997) Music increases satisfaction in elderly outpatients undergoing cataract surgery. *Canadian Journal of Anaesthesia*, 44(1), 43–8.

Daykin, N., Byrne, E., Soteriou, T. and O'Connor, S. (2010) Using arts to enhance mental healthcare environments: findings from qualitative research. *Arts and Health*, 2(1), 33–46.

Daykin, N., Mansfield, L., Meads, C., Julier, G., Tomlinson, A., Payne, A., Grigsby, D., Lane, J., D'Innocenzo, G., Burnett, A., Kay, T., Dolan, P., Stefano, T. and Victor, C. (2018) What works for wellbeing? A systematic review of wellbeing outcomes for music and singing in adults. *Perspectives in Public Health*, 138(1), 39–46.

Deci, E.L. and Ryan, R.M. (2012) Self-determination theory. In Van Lange, P.A.M., Kruglanski, A.W. and Higgins, E.T. eds., *Handbook of theories of social psychology*. London: Sage, vol. 1, 416–36.

Devlin, A.S. and Arneill, A.B. (2003) Health Care Environments and Patient Outcomes: A Review of the Literature. *Environment and Behavior*, 35(5), 665–94, available: https://doi.org/10.1177/0013916503255102.

Dingle, G.A., Clift, S., Finn, S., Gilbert, R., Groarke, J.M., Irons, J.Y., Bartoli, A.J., Lamont, A., Launay, J., Martin, E.S., Moss, H., Sanfilippo, K.R., Shipton, M., Stewart, L., Talbot, S., Tarrant, M., Tip, L. and Williams, E.J. (2019) An Agenda for Best Practice Research on Group Singing, Health, and Well-Being. *Music & Science*, 2, available: http://dx.doi.org/10.1177/2059204319861719.

Dose, L. (2006) National Network for the Arts in Health: lessons learned from six years of work. *The Journal of the Royal Society for the Promotion of Health*, 126(3), 110–12.

Drahota, A., Ward, D., Mackenzie, H., Stores, R., Higgins, B., Gal, D. and Dean Taraneh, P. (2012) Sensory environment on health-related outcomes of hospital patients. *Cochrane Database of Systematic Reviews*.

Fancourt, D. and Perkins, R. (2017) Associations between singing to babies and symptoms of postnatal depression, wellbeing, self-esteem and mother-infant bond. *Public Health*, 145, 149–52, available: http://dx.doi.org/10.1016/j.puhe.2017.01.016.

Fancourt, D., Williamon, A., Carvalho, L., Steptoe, A., Dow, R. and Lewis, I. (2016) Singing modulates mood, stress, cortisol, cytokine and neuropeptide activity in cancer patients and carers. *ecancer*, 10(631), available: http://dx.doi.org/10.3332/ecancer.2016.631.

Fidler, H. and Mikszka, P. (2020) Music interventions and pain: an integrative review and analysis of recent literature. *Approaches: An Interdisciplinary Journal of Music Therapy*, 12(1), available: https://approaches.gr.

Fitzgerald, D. and Callard, F. (2015) *Rethinking interdisciplinarity across the social sciences and neurosciences*. Basingstoke: Palgrave Macmillan.

Fitzpatrick, K., Moss, H. and Harmon, D. (2019) .Music in the chronic pain experience: An Investigation into the Use of Music and Music therapy by Patients and Staff at a Hospital Outpatient Pain Clinic. *Music and Medicine*, 11, 6–22.

Flower C. and Meadows G. (2019) *'Music while you wait': developing music therapy in maternity care*. London: Chelsea and Westminster Hospital NHS Foundation Trust.

Flower, C. and Watts, G. (2018) *'Music While You Wait': the impact of music therapy in maternity services at Chelsea and Westminster Hospital (2017–2018)*. London: Chelsea and Westminster Hospital NHS Foundation Trust.

Flower, C. and Watts, G. (2019) *'Music While You Wait': the impact of music therapy in maternity services at Chelsea and Westminster Hospital (2017–2018)*. London: Chelsea and Westminster Hospital NHS Foundation Trust.

Garza-Villarreal, E.A., Wilson, A.D., Vase, L., Brattico, E., Barrios, F.A., Jensen, T.S., Romero-Romo, J.I. and Vuust, P. (2014) Music reduces pain and increases functional mobility in fibromyalgia. *Frontiers in Psychology*, 5, available: http://dx.doi.org/10.3389/fpsyg.2014.00090.

Gaut, B. and McIver Lopes, D. eds. (2005) *The Routledge companion to aesthetics*, 2nd ed. Abingdon: Routledge.

Gleeson, S. (2019) *Constellations: reflections from life*. London: Picador.

Gold, C., Heldal Tor, O., Dahle, T. and Wigram, T. (2005) Music therapy for schizophrenia or schizophrenia-like illnesses. *Cochrane Database of Systematic Reviews*.

Goldenberg, R.B. (2017) Singing Lessons for Respiratory Health: A Literature Review. *J Voice*, 32(1), 85–94, doi: 10.1016/j.jvoice.2017.03.021.

Graham, G. (1997) *Philosophy of the arts: an introduction to aesthetics*. London: Routledge.

Grover, C., Mackasey, E., Cook, E., Tremblay, L. and Loiselle, C.G. (2018). Patient-reported care domains that enhance the experience of "being known" in an ambulatory cancer care centre. *Canadian Oncology Nursing Journal*, 28(3), 166–71, available: www.ncbi.nlm.nih.gov/pmc/articles/PMC6516925/.

Health Service Executive (2019) *Postpartum psychosis*, available: www2.hse.ie/conditions/mental-health/postnatal-depression/postpartum-psychosis.html.

Huisman, E.R.C.M., Morales, E., van Hoof, J. and Kort, H.S.M. (2012) Healing environment: A review of the impact of physical environmental factors on users. *Building and Environment*, 58, 70–80, available: http://dx.doi.org/https://doi.org/10.1016/j.buildenv.2012.06.016.

Irons, J.Y., Kenny, D.T. and Chang. A.B. (2010) Singing for children and adults with bronchiectasis. *Cochrane Database of Systematic Reviews*, available: http://doi:10.1002/14651858.CD007729.pub2.

Irons, J.Y., Petocz, P., Kenny, D.T. and Chang, A.B. (2019) Singing as an adjunct therapy for children and adults with cystic fibrosis. *Cochrane Database of Systematic Reviews*, available: www.cochranelibrary.com/cdsr/doi/10.1002/14651858.CD008036.pub5/full.

Jeffries S. and Groves N. (2014) Hans Ulrich Obrist: the art of curation. *The Guardian*, available: www.theguardian.com/artanddesign/2014/mar/23/hans-ulrich-obrist-art-curator.

Jespersen, K.V., Koenig, J., Jennum, P. and Vuust, P. (2015) Music for insomnia in adults. *Cochrane Database of Systematic Reviews*, available: http://dx.doi.org/10.1002/14651858.CD010459.pub2.

Jonas, W.B. and Chez, R.A. (2004) Toward Optimal Healing Environments in Health Care. *The Journal of Alternative and Complementary Medicine*, 10 (supplement 1), S-1–S-6, available: www.liebertpub.com/doi/10.1089/acm.2004.10.S-1.

Kieran, M. (2005) Value of art. In Gaut, B. and McIver Lopes, D., eds., *The Routledge companion to aesthetics*, 2nd ed. Abingdon: Routledge, 293–307.

Kilroy, A., Garner, C., Parkinson, C., Kagan, C. and Senior, P. (2007) *Towards Transformation: Exploring the impact of culture, creativity and the arts on health and wellbeing. A consultation report for the critical friends event*, Manchester: Arts for Health, Manchester Metropolitan University.

Kirklin, D. and Richardson, R. eds. (2003) *The Healing Environment: Without and Within*, London: Royal College of Physicians.

Laopaiboon, M., Lumbiganon, P., Martis, R., Vatanasapt, P. and Somjaivong, B. (2009) Music during caesarean section under regional anaesthesia for improving maternal and infant outcomes. *Cochrane Database of Systematic Reviews*, available: http://dx.doi.org/10.1002/14651858.CD006914.pub2.

Lawson, B. (2001) *The language of space*. Oxford: Architectural Press.

Lawson, B. (2003) Healing Architecture. *Arts and Health*, 2(2), 95–108.

Lee, J.H. (2016) The Effects of Music on Pain: A Meta-Analysis. *Journal of Music Therapy*, 53(4), 430–77.

Levitin, D.J. (2008) *This is your brain on music: understanding a human obsession*. London: Atlantic.

MacDonald, R.A.R., Hargreaves, D.J. and Miell, D. (2002) *Musical identities*. Oxford: Oxford University Press.

MacDonald, R.A.R., Kreutz, G. and Mitchell, L. (2012) *Music, health, and wellbeing*. Oxford: Oxford University Press.

Magee, W.L., Clark, I., Tamplin, J. and Bradt, J. (2017) Music interventions for acquired brain injury. *Cochrane Database of Systematic Reviews*, available: https://doi.org/10.1002/14651858.CD006787.pub3.

Mandoki, K. (2007) *Everyday aesthetics: prosaics, the play of culture and social identities*. London: Ashgate.

McNamara, R.J., Epsley, C., Coren, E. and McKeough, Z.J. (2017) Singing for adults with chronic obstructive pulmonary disease. *Cochrane Database of Systematic Reviews*, available: www.cochranelibrary.com/cdsr/doi/10.1002/14651858.CD012296.pub2/full.

Mitchell, L.A. and MacDonald, R.A. (2006) An experimental investigation of the effects of preferred and relaxing music listening on pain perception. *Journal of Music Therapy*, 43(4), 295–316.

Morris, D. (2008) Narrative medicines: challenge and resistance. *The Permanente Journal*, 12, 88–96.

Moss, H., Donnellan, C. and O'Neill, D. (2015) Hospitalization and aesthetic health in older adults. *Journal of the American Medical Directors Association*, 16(2), 173.e11–173.e16, available: http://dx.doi.org/10.1016/j.jamda.2014.10.019.

Moss, H. and O'Neill, D. (2014a) The aesthetic and cultural interests of patients attending an acute hospital – a phenomenological study. *Journal of Advanced Nursing*, 70(1), 121–9, available: https://doi.org/10.1111/jan.12175.

Moss, H. and O'Neill, D. (2014b) The art of medicine: Aesthetic deprivation in clinical settings. *The Lancet*, 383(9922), 1032–3, available: https://doi.org/10.1016/S0140-6736(14)60507-9.

Moss, H., Lynch, J. and O'Donoghue, J. (2017a) Exploring the perceived health benefits of singing in a choir: an international cross-sectional mixed-methods study. *Perspectives in Public Health*, 138, 160–68, available: http://dx.doi.org/DOI: 10.1177/1757913917739652.

Moss, H., Lynch, J. and O'Donoghue, J. (2017b) *Sing yourself better: the health and wellbeing benefits of singing in a choir*. Report. Irish World Academy of Music and Dance: University of Limerick.

Moss, H., Nolan, E. and O'Neill, D. (2007) A cure for the soul? The benefit of live music in the general hospital. *Irish Medical Journal*, 100(10), 636–8.

Moss, H. and O'Donoghue, J. (2018) *Sing while you work – the well-being benefits of workplace choirs*. Limerick: University of Limerick, available: http://hdl.handle.net/10344/7257.

Moss, H. and O'Neill, D. (2014) The aesthetic and cultural interests of patients attending an acute hospital – a phenomenological study. *Journal of Advanced Nursing*, 70(1), 121–9.

Moss, H. and O'Neill, D. (2019) The role of the curator in modern hospitals: a transcontinental perspective. *Journal of Medical Humanities*, 40(1), 85–100, available: https://doi.org/10.1007/s10912-016-94.23-3.

Notarangelo, A. (2019) Music therapy and spiritual care: Music as spiritual support in a hospital environment. *Approaches: An Interdisciplinary Journal of Music Therapy*, Special Issue 11.

O'Neill, A. and Moss, H. (2015) A community art therapy group for adults with chronic pain. *Art Therapy*, 32(4), 158–67, available: https://doi.org/10.1080/07421656.2015.1091642.

O'Neill, D., Jenkins, E., Mawhinney, R., Cosgrave, E., O'Mahony, S., Guest, C. and Moss, H. (2016) Rethinking the medical in the medical humanities. *Medical Humanities*, 42(2), 109–14, available: http://dx.doi.org/10.1136/medhum-2015–010831.

Parsons, G. (2010) *Beauty and public policy*. London: Commission for Architecture and the Built Environment.

Pavlicevic, M. (2003) *Groups in music: strategies from music therapy*. London: Jessica Kingsley.

Robins, S. (2019) *Bird's eye view: stories of a life lived in health care*. Vancouver: Bird Communications.

Saito, Y. (2008) *Everyday aesthetics*. Oxford: Oxford University Press.

Sato, Y. (2011) 'Musical Life Review in Hospice', *Music Therapy Perspectives*, 29(1), 31–8, available: https://doi.org/10.1093/mtp/29.1.31.

Sarkamo, T., Tervaniemi, M., Laitinen, S., Forsblom, A., Soinila, S., Mikkonen, M., Autti, T., Silvennoinen, H., Erkkila, J., Laine, M., Peretz, I. and Hietanen,

M. (2008) Music listening enhances cognitive recovery and mood after middle cerebral artery stroke. *Brain*, 131, 866–76.

Scott, J., Cork, R., Z, P., Hall, A., Mercier, A., Ferry, D., Saull, G. and Khan, L. (2019) The Healing Arts: the arts project at Chelsea and Westminster Hospital. London: Unicorn.

Selle, E.W. and Silverman, M.J. (2017) A randomized feasibility study on the effects of music therapy in the form of patient-preferred live music on mood and pain in patients on a cardiovascular unit. *Arts & Health*, 9(3), 213–23, available: https://doi.org/10.1080/17533015.2017.1334678.

Slettebø, Å., Sæteren, B., Caspari, S., Lohne, V., Rehnsfeldt, A.W., Heggestad, A.K.T., Lillestø, B., Høy, B., Råholm, M.B., Lindwall, L., Aasgaard, T. and Nåden, D. (2017) The significance of meaningful and enjoyable activities for nursing home resident's experiences of dignity. *Scandinavian Journal of Caring Sciences*, 31(4), 718–26, available: http://dx.doi.org/10.1111/scs.12386.

Tolstoy, L. (1930) *What is art?* Oxford: Oxford University Press.

Smith, C.A., Collins, C.T., Cyna, A.M. and Crowther, C.A. (2006) Complementary and alternative therapies for pain management in labour. *Cochrane Database of Systematic Reviews*, available: http://dx.doi.org/10.1002/14651858.CD003521.pub2.

Ulrich, R. (1992) How design impacts wellness. *Healthcare Forum Journal*, 35(5), 20–25.

Ulrich R and Gilpin L (2003) Healing arts: nutrition for the soul. In Frampton, S., Gilpin, L. and Charmel, P.A., eds., *Putting patients first: designing and practicing patient-centered care*. San Francisco: Jossey-Bass, 117–46.

Van der Steen, J.T., Smaling, H.J.A., Van der Wouden, J.C., Bruinsma, M.S., Scholten, R. and Vink, A.C. (2018) Music-based therapeutic interventions for people with dementia. *Cochrane Database of Systematic Reviews*.

Welch, G., Howard, D. and Nix, J. (2019) *The Oxford handbook of singing*. Oxford: Oxford University Press.

Wood, J., Sandford, S. and Bailey, E. (2016) 'The whole is greater'. Developing music therapy services in the National Health Service: a case study revisited. *British Journal of Music Therapy*, 30, 36–46.

5   Polyphony

Issues of professionalism and working as a team

Aesthetic enrichment needs to be an organisation wide concern. Clinicians and managers need to attend to engagement in arts, cultural and leisure pursuits for best results. Healthcare staff are often time-poor, concerned with client crises, costs, discharge rates, paperwork and volume of clients. It can be difficult to think about 'frivolous embellishments' such as music therapy or visual art in the ward, and people only gain access to the supports possible through the arts when the music therapist or arts professional is integrated into the team throughout the care pathway (Twyford and Watson 2008). Full integration with the healthcare team makes a difference, and this chapter explores professional issues in caring through music.

Returning to Claire's story

This chapter begins with a postscript to Claire's story (detailed in Chapter 4). Claire benefitted from one drop-in music therapy session while she was an in-patient in a mental healthcare facility. This musical care was ad hoc, spontaneous and happened purely by accident. Nonetheless, I believe this interaction offered Claire a positive and hopeful moment in a time of despair and allowed her to express her love and gratitude for her husband who was caring for their new baby while she was sick. The musical care Claire received was limited. With improved teamwork and interdisciplinary communication, she could have engaged in further music therapy sessions and continued this useful work. This chapter reviews and recommends how to work well with the professional team to ensure quality integration of music in healthcare settings.

In ongoing music therapy with Claire, we might have recorded her song, carried out some family bonding sessions with her children and/or partner as part of her rehabilitation and supported her recovery as she journeyed from acute inpatient crisis to outpatient care, as she returned to home in her role as a mother and partner. I may have referred her to my colleagues running community music groups or community song writing classes. Issues of organisational culture made this impossible. I was a visiting, sessional music therapist, not linked adequately with the clinical team and therefore had limited capacity to recommend she received individual music therapy or to offer continued work as an outpatient or in her own home. Similarly, a lack of clear networks between musicians working in health and wellbeing contexts also made this impossible. This chapter explores issues amongst musicians in health settings and between clinical professionals, both of which can hamper music care initiatives.

Music in healthcare settings: a variety of professionals working alongside one another

It is impossible to prioritise one creative arts activity over another. For example, music therapy, music performance and music listening are equally valuable, as is access to reading material, film or live theatre performance. What matters, in my experience, is that the creative activity is matched to the personal preference of the person receiving care (in other words what they need or want at a particular time) and ties in with reflection on their needs by clinicians, family and artists involved in their care. This may not be adequately considered if focused on ensuring standardised delivery of interventions.

The context of the healthcare setting, the phase of treatment or illness, the social context of the individual and their preferences must determine what is offered and provided by arts practitioners. The expert musician, working in hospital, can bring knowledge and experience to the situation, perhaps offering opportunities that the person has never imagined or experienced.

Unfortunately, arts in healthcare is a splintered profession and music may more likely be offered to reluctant service users or imposed upon those receiving care. Arts therapists, arts and health practitioners, performers, community artists and creative technologists are separated by artificial divisions and insecurities. Few health service managers have a fully thought out rationale for arts therapies, or community arts, or a performance programme in their nursing home or hospital. An ad hoc approach is more common, with practitioners often competing for funds for the arts and the one that started there first tending to determine the culture.

As hospital Arts Manager, I developed a new approach to arts and health practice, in which I determined that the term 'arts and health' referred to *all* arts related activity that existed in our hospital. This perspective aimed to counter the artificial and defensive barriers constructed between practitioners and professional groups within the field, encourage greater respect and understanding between arts practitioners and assist in identifying training for the various arts professionals. My experience has taught me that unhelpful assumptions currently exist between arts therapists and arts and health practitioners, and these need to be challenged. Competition for funding, rigidity in professional specialisms and political priorities dominate the field.

For example, some artists do not recognise the artistic capabilities of arts therapists. Similarly, some arts therapists view all creative work by untrained therapists to be suspicious, dangerous, inappropriate or unsafe. Arts and health funding is often available only to artists using a participatory or collaborative framework rather than a therapy perspective. On the other hand, some health services employ arts therapists on salary scales as clinical professionals, whereas artists are left to fight for grants or bursaries and sustained practice can be difficult to establish.[1]

As a clinical supervisor I spent many hours with music therapists defining and re-defining how they see their role and remit in their particular clinical setting, whilst simultaneously engaging with funding bodies where only participatory or collaborative arts projects were eligible for arts and health funding. Similarly, I engaged in professional activities in medical humanities, arts and health and arts therapies groupings and found overlaps throughout, for example in the areas of singing and health or museum education programmes and curatorship. I experienced that all activities and approaches offer specific benefits to service users at particular times in their journey towards improved health and well-being, and all can cause harm if delivered by poorly prepared practitioners. Confusion and difficulties exist in the current ad hoc approach to funding, employment conditions and practice. Overall, my impression, after years in the field, was that the service user's arts preferences and needs were being neglected, due to arts practitioners focus on their own practice needs and recognition of their identity within the diverse field.

Music and health: working at the edges

Kira Tozer of the Arts Health Network Canada gives a compelling definition of arts and health (Tozer 2015):

> Arts & Health is an umbrella term that includes [these] pursuits: bringing visual arts, music, performances and art-making opportunities into healthcare environments; the creative arts therapies like music therapy, dance therapy, art therapy; community arts projects that address health or social problems faced by a group of people; arts-based health research; arts-based health communication; using the arts

in the education of health care professionals etcetera. The arts and health can intersect in many different ways, with different aims and outcomes. The arts can help us to understand, communicate and cope with various experiences of human illness – be it our own or a loved one's, a service user's or a provider's. The arts help to reconnect us with the human element of health and health care.

This definition sums up my approach to music in healthcare spaces, a broad church that includes any way we use music to further our health and well-being, including the many different approaches used in healthcare spaces.

The important feature of the diagram in Figure 5.1 is that 'music and health' is no longer a term understood as *not arts therapies* or *participative arts* or *collaborative arts*. For example, receptive (i.e. listening to live and recorded music) and background music are as important as participatory and therapeutic activities. For some health service users, normalised access to music activities that they enjoy will be more important than engaging in therapy or workshops. We are eager, as professional musicians, to emphasise active participation over receptive arts and this is reflected in significant gaps in the literature about the health and well-being benefits of receptive arts (Moss

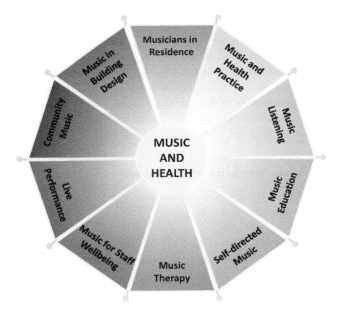

Figure 5.1 Music and health: a new model of practice (Moss 2016)[2]

et al. 2012). As one clinician observed, 'Most of us go to concerts or recitals, but for some reason we always offer service users a workshop'.

Unfortunately, this model of working alongside each other as musicians in healthcare is great in theory but rarely practiced in reality. The field of music and health is diverse, with no comprehensive view of music and health, standards of practice or agreed training. Anyone can set up as a musician working in healthcare settings and quality can be variable. This is not safe for service users. Music therapists are significantly further along this developmental journey with standards of practice and professional regulation in some countries (WFMT 2017). The profession of music therapy has worked hard to establish itself, but part of this work has involved adopting a model in which it *narrowed its practice and theory in pursuit of the golden brick of medical and statutory legitimacy* (Ansdell 2014; Murphy 2018). The circular nature of the diagram in Figure 5.1 indicates that each approach is equally valuable. What is essential is careful curation and high quality so that each activity, intervention or approach is chosen for a specific reason at a specific time, ideally by a sensitive, expert professional or stakeholder group.

Early in my career I realised that different phases of hospital care bring with them different needs. Feedback from hospital service users indicated that when you are acutely ill, dealing with emergency or surgery, you are happy to 'park' your interests – you don't expect to see family, friends or continue your normal interests. You don't even feel like reading a book. If you do, the arts intervention can only be a moment in the day, albeit an important one, of hope and/or beauty amongst the fear and confusion of being acutely ill. Acute pain is rarely a time for a Tolstoy novel or a Mahler symphony, often we feel more inclined to flick the pages of a magazine or listen to something 'easy' which takes less mental effort as our body is expending huge amounts of energy on coping with sickness. There is a creative tension between the low expectations of hospital stakeholders regarding music in the environment and international evidence of benefit. Music experts in healthcare settings need to keep a watchful eye on international practice and research in order to be able to make positive, creative suggestions that are currently unimaginable.

Music and health: a continuum of practice

To date research has focused on participatory music-making rather than receptive and performative music in healthcare spaces. Little work has been done to identify the specific skill sets required for different musical activities and interventions. This gap informed my second diagram (Figure 5.2).

In this continuum, all types of music practice are equally valuable. The continuum represents the skills required and the client needs. Whilst there

Music and health – a continuum of practice

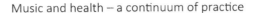

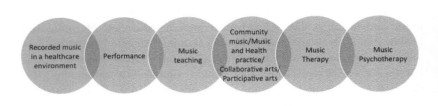

Figure 5.2 Music and health: a continuum of practice (Moss 2016)

is fluidity and movement between roles, the continuum indicates that extra training or specialised skills may be required at either end of the continuum. The aim of this diagram is to challenge the status quo that sees music and health emerging as a predominantly participative arts field, to the exclusion of other approaches, and to return to the idea of music and health as a broad field that interacts with health and well-being in myriad ways.

Jane's story: is it music therapy or music and health practice?

Jane, a professional musician visited children in hospital in a large acute teaching hospital where I was the arts manager. Every week she specialised in singing lullabies to sick infants, engaging the children and their parents or guardians in improvisational music-making. The aim of the session was to soothe children in hospital, make their hospital stay a more positive experience, offer positive distraction from pain, and to encourage the parents/ guardians to sing with their babies. Are these clinical or musical aims? Or perhaps educational aims? Is this best provided by a music therapist, a music and health practitioner or a professional performing musician? What training is needed to provide this session effectively?

Jane identifies herself as a musician, performing for children and parents and not engaging in therapeutic activity, despite contributing to treatment and helping children to cope with pain. In identifying her training needs, we decided she would benefit from mentoring, training on childhood illness and childhood bereavement and both personal development and self-care input. Alongside Jane's programme, the hospital schoolteacher engaged a music teacher to run sessions in the school room while Tom, the music therapist in the hospital, also provided individual music therapy to children with diabetes.

At the same time, a community musician from a respected children's arts charity made contact to develop a community music engagement in the hospital. How do we manage these different activities and interventions in a coherent way and how does Jane maintain her professional identity and expertise alongside the many other practitioners in this space?

'We need some orientation tools, as the field of music, culture and health is rapidly growing and becoming potentially confusing' (Bonde 2011). Jane's example serves to demonstrate the complexities and crowdedness of working as a musician in a healthcare setting. My approach to solving this conundrum can be broken down into the following five recommendations.

1) Develop a clear vision, strategy and policy for music in hospital. As Director of Arts and Health I brought together all stakeholders to devise the arts and health programme at the hospital and to tease out how the various musicians might work alongside one another. I insisted upon quarterly team meetings of all artists working at the hospital, whatever their approach or professional identity. At the meeting common ground was explored and training delivered in areas of shared practice (for example, ethical issues common to all practitioners, developing creative and flexible responses, training on self-care).

2) Keep the service user at the centre of decision-making. The needs and wishes of service users was at the core of team planning. Communication with clinicians is important too, as they can speak to the care needs of the people they serve. For example, the consultant geriatricians, clinical nurse specialists and speech and language therapists for people with dementia at the hospital were integral to discussion of which arts programmes should be provided in the older age care wards, with music therapy, visual art groups, bedside art, dancer in residence and live performance forming the varied programme at one time.

3) Model an equality of respect and value. All artists received training, funding opportunities to attend conferences and supervision time from senior practitioners and managers. Due to the large size of the team, I introduced a new structure with two senior practitioners who helped me to supervise the arts team. These two people were an Art Therapist and a Visual Artist in Residence. There was no hierarchy here between them, both were rewarded for their fine practice and senior expertise and they took on a team of junior artists and arts therapists to train and support.

4) Reclaim 'arts and health'. I insisted that arts and health must be a broad umbrella term and not be hijacked by one or other profession.

5) Clear aims and objectives. Everyone in the team must be able to give a clear rationale as to why they are providing an activity, its' potential

benefit and what evidence there is that service users and clinicians welcome this initiative. The success of our team lay, I believe, in everyone being clear as to the aim(s) of their work and where their professional boundaries lay.

Two other models are worth noting here. MacDonald (2013) and Bonde (2011) describe valuable models of working in the music and health field.

Steven's story

Steven's story illustrates the role of many different music professionals in one person's care journey. I met Steven when he was an outpatient attending a mental health facility in London. He was a single man aged twenty-four who lived at home with his parents and was in a long-term relationship. He was referred to me by his Psychiatrist and Art Therapist. I worked with Steven once a week for a year, until I suggested termination of music therapy and referral on to psychotherapy and community music.

Until the age of twenty-two, Steven played bass guitar in a band. The band had recently released a moderately successful album and were gaining notice. They had been asked to play at some significant gigs and it was believed that they were on the cusp of 'making it'. Steven was walking home late at night and was hit by a truck. He suffered a serious brain injury and spent five months in hospital, first having emergency brain surgery and later receiving painstaking rehabilitation in a neuro rehabilitation hospital to regain function. He spent time in intensive care, where his family were told to expect the worse of outcomes and described his recovery as a miracle. When I met him, he was living at home with his parents and attending the community mental health team. He was also receiving support from a national voluntary organisation for people with acquired brain injury.

Steven made an excellent recovery from his injury and exceeded all forecasts for his future. His cognitive and physical function was excellent with no sustained disability in these areas. He was referred due to irritability, verbal aggression, depression and lethargy. He was being supported through mental health services for these issues.

Steven was referred to music therapy for three reasons: (1) to re-activate his strong interest in music to meet his rehabilitation goals; (2) to pursue and improve his guitar playing as a potential work and/or leisure activity; (3) to improve his low motivation and energy levels; and (4) to lift his mood. Steven found it very hard to get up and out of the house in time for appointments or to see through any commitments to weekly activities. His hygiene was poor and his motivation was minimal. However, he was keen to attend individual music therapy and from the first week was highly motivated and engaged.

Music therapists often witness an otherwise unmotivated or unresponsive person reacting strongly to music. Music stimulates several regions of the brain simultaneously and can produce quite unexpected and striking responses (Levitin 2008). The motivation afforded by musical activities can assist people to re-engage in community activities (for example choirs for people with dementia). The film of Senator Gabby Giffords illustrates this phenomenon.

> Listen and watch online 5.1: Gabby Giffords finds her voice through music therapy www.youtube.com/watch?v=tiJ9X_wLSWM

Steven attended music therapy regularly. Taking a psychodynamic music therapy approach, I discovered there were several interesting strands to the work. Firstly, as the music therapist I regularly felt drained of energy, tired and even sleepy in the sessions and began to realise that this was countertransference. Steven sometimes came late or sent a message that he would not attend the session. I had to work very hard to maintain energy for the sessions and to organise them.

Steven described how his mother had to look after him 'as if he was a baby again' when he first had his brain injury (feeding him, bathing him, clothing him). Whilst he was now independent, he still lived in his parents' home and had no plans to separate and live independently. There was a sense of his mother and him being closely bonded, but perhaps also co-dependent as both were dealing with serious health issues themselves. At one point in the work, I suggested that Steven choose an instrument to represent his mother, father and himself and we improvised various combinations of these dyad relationships. The resulting improvisations gave Steven clarity about the relationships with his parents. Until this time there had been extensive talking about his parents but little insight into the dynamics of the relationships. Music played a key role in bringing insight to Steven and provided a way for him to reflect with me about his goals, hopes and limitations. In music therapy I became aware of a strong desire to 'mother' Steven also. I began to invest too heavily in his progress and his needs and it was only by attending clinical supervision that I recognised the transference and was able to support Steven without over-protecting him. For example, I began planning to take Steven to a community music session to help him make the move from therapy to community engaged music-making. On reflection with my clinical supervisor and mentor, I realised that it was not normal for me to consider doing this for a client, so why was I getting so involved and planning to spend an evening accompanying Steven to this activity when he was a grown man who was quite capable of organising himself to attend if he wanted to?

Steven appeared to idolize me and loved music therapy. The improvisations we created in the sessions were musically sophisticated and Steven was always enthusiastic about how excellent music therapy was. I also found the improvisation very rewarding as Steven was an accomplished musician. I used my psychodynamic training to maintain an appropriate professional boundary (issues such as how to deal with Steven wanting to hug me goodbye and whether to swap mobile phone numbers were discussed and reflected upon). Clinical supervision proved vital here in maintaining a supportive but boundaried relationship.

One of Steven's aims for music therapy was to work towards re-establishing a link with musicians, and eventually to join a band again. A step on the way was to attend a community music group in the local arts centre. I referred him to this group. Community music played a crucial part in Steven's rehabilitation and development of his new musical identity. Steven attended drumming circles in his local arts centre for the year following therapy. He worked on developing his ability to perform again and to attend performances and festivals as he had prior to his injury.

Steven's friends also played a significant role in his journey. His contacts in the music world offered occasional opportunities to jam together and try out music again. This was informal but critical to building confidence and overcoming the lethargy that was part of his illness. Finally, listening to music was a constant friend during Steven's illness. He listened to music every day. One cannot underestimate the role receptive music played in his care, during both the long days in hospital and when he was at home, unable to motivate himself to go out. When he finished therapy, I also recommended engaging in music education, as I thought that taking lessons with an expert bass player might ignite Steven's love for his instrument once again.

The person at the centre of this story had a massive, shocking, sudden trauma in his life, which changed the course of his life and his identity. He lost the support and belonging he had enjoyed as a successful member of a band. He had no other obvious career routes and was currently not earning. His needs spanned his mental health, social connection, rebuilding his identity, working through emotional issues, post-traumatic stress and creativity. This is a complex case and I hope it gives an example of how different approaches played an important part in his recovery, at different times. An experienced professional will recognise the limits of their approach and interventions and be open to other methods. After a year of therapy I referred Steven on to a psychotherapist as he was increasingly using music therapy for verbal processing. I felt I had reached the limit of my skill in this area and that he would benefit from talking therapy. Steven had also engaged with the drumming circle at this stage and I believed he was able to fulfil his musical needs in community music activities. Unfortunately, Steven continued to struggle with low motivation and lethargy and so this positive story has some caveats. He continued to struggle to achieve his aims but music continued to be an important source of positive outlet for him. Steven benefitted from music therapy, community music, playing bass alone and with friends and listening to music. At least four of the music approaches in my model were relevant and important to Steven.

Leah's story

Leah was a violinist who offered to perform in her local hospital as she was interested in this area of work. Mary was a nurse manager working in the High Dependency Unit who agreed to have her play once a week. Leah joined the hospital volunteer programme with minimal training or induction. Mary invited Leah to play music on the ward just outside the nurses' station where several people in single rooms could listen. One of the service users was Keith, a very frail older person with pneumonia and other health complications. As Leah played, Keith showed signs of deterioration in his vital signs and some distress. Mary closed his bedroom door to shut out the music as it did not appear to be having a positive effect on Keith and instructed Leah to play more gently. Keith's condition stabilised. Mary made the decision to conclude the music and move Leah to the far end of the corridor. Mary had not consulted the hospital music therapist for advice as she was employed only to work in the psychiatry and paediatric wards. In later years, the musician volunteers were offered training and induction centrally by the senior music therapist, who vetted potential volunteers and offered support, supervision and liaison to ensure that live music performance in ward areas was appropriately curated.

Interdisciplinarity

In my experience the best music and health projects are those which are interdisciplinary, between clinicians, musicians and service users. The isolated musician is unsupported, at risk of doing harm, may not be able to use music's potential and may burn out very quickly. Managers and clinicians who instigate music without taking advice from musicians may equally do harm or fail to explore music's potential clinical and therapeutic reach. Without service user involvement, music programmes are often ill-judged, of little effect or worse injurious. A perfect example is the willing but limited local choir who come in to sing Christmas carols. The clinician thinks this is a wonderful idea and invites them in, but the music therapist working in the ward hears them and realises with horror that their music is aesthetically poor and out of tune. The service user swears under their breath at having to listen to yet more carol singers! Another example is the musician who has a great idea for a performance project where she will write new songs with input from service users. She fails to engage with the clinicians and managers and only upon starting to work realises that the time of day she has chosen clashes with important clinical sessions and is a time when many service users are tired. She has also failed to investigate the needs of service users and staff, so missed the opportunity to offer staff a music session for their well-being and to meet the expressed desire of service users to form a choir for peer support. Fitzgerald and Callard (2015) explore the benefits and issues of interdisciplinarity in detail.

Staff in hospital act as gatekeepers of the arts. Nurse managers on wards either allow or block access to music for service users. They have strong opinions about the arts and refer service users to arts services or discourage contact. For example, the ward manager generally decides whether music in the ward is positive, as it will encourage social activity, or will be a noise disturbance and should be curbed. In my work, collaboration and support was needed for any musician to implement a programme successfully in the hospital. The greatest opportunities came from collaboration and inter-disciplinary working. Where I partnered with a doctor, speech and language therapist, nurse specialist or occupational therapist to design a programme, the results were more effective than trying to instigate change alone. Where this collaboration involved service users the results were sometimes extraordinary (Crawford 2015; Crawford, Brown and Charise 2020).

In the hospitals, nursing homes and day centres I worked in, the common practice was (and still is) to prioritise medication, feeding, washing, dressing and medical treatments and tests, and when all that was done, to leave a person sitting comfortably in a chair until the next intervention is required. 'Activity coordinators' are now popular posts within health settings, their remit to provide meaningful activity for service users. This is a great attempt at considering the cultural and leisure pursuits of service users, but often little budget or specialist expertise is provided in this area, and the result can be low quality activities offered on a shoestring through volunteerism. In my experience, activity coordinators are expected to perform miracles, namely to provide a meaningful programme of activities to people in their care without a budget or resources to provide for specialist input nor the training to fully assess the individual needs of each person in their care.

As a musician, music therapist and curator of all art forms within a hospital, I began to build a team around me to address the need for beauty, choice and control over the aesthetic environment of the hospital. It was no good to stay in my silo of 'music' or even worse 'music therapy'. I had to start with what would help the service users. Ross and McSherry (2018) recommend all clinicians ask two simple but profound questions to guide all their work in healthcare spaces: 'What is important to you right now?' and 'How can I help?'

Natural partners in hospitals include doctors, psychologists, nurses, occupational therapists and pastoral care specialists. Many use music in their own practice. Anyone interested in quality of care in addition to treatment and cure is an ally in hospital settings. During my research and practice, I surveyed one hundred and fifty people aged over 65 about their arts and cultural interests before, during and after hospital. The vast majority of participants identified as active singers, painters or dancers before they were admitted to hospital, but not one could continue their arts interests in hospital. Many did not even consider it a possibility to bring in their favourite music from home, or their paints or their guitar. Hospital was not a space for this. Without collaboration with clinical colleagues we will never be able to introduce normal aesthetic and cultural interests, let alone develop clinically specific interventions. In another older age ward, I provided music therapy (individual and group therapy) but increasingly felt uncomfortable with the atmosphere in the day area of the ward. I introduced both an open singing group (for staff, family members and service users) to lift the mood on the ward and set about purchasing listening devices for use by individuals on the ward to listen to their favourite music. In another ward, I worked with end of life specialists to create a quiet space where families could gather during the end of life vigil, and we used colour, art and music to create a caring, restful space for people to base themselves during this difficult time.

A successful recent project has involved a Consultant Anaesthetist working at an acute hospital, me as music researcher, and a PhD student who is qualified as both a community musician and a music therapist. Together we have developed a programme of work which has included exploring live and recorded music in the waiting room of the pain clinic, documenting the musical interests of service users with particular attention to how they use music to cope with living with chronic pain, a qualitative study of individual music therapy with ten participants, and a mixed method study of group music therapy in a community setting. The strength of this team is the openness of all to work together and develop (Fitzpatrick et al. 2019).

> We need an epistemological culture of *filoxenia* (etymology from the Greek *filo* [= love] + *xenos* [= stranger]); a spirit of openness, trust and generosity…. instead of being uninvited or misunderstood guests in each other's disciplinary discourses [we must] collaborate as partners and equally important co-creators of this interdisciplinary environment.
> (Tsiris and Ansdell 2020)

Another successful project is called *The Dance Back Home*. Dancer in residence Ailish Claffey worked with film maker and artist Deirdre Glenfield to create a 15-minute film of her work with older people in the Age Related Health Care Unit at Tallaght Hospital, Dublin. The resulting film shows collaboration in action between doctors, physiotherapists, dancer, music therapist, nurses, nursing assistants, service users, family carers and artists. This beautiful film captures the success of interdisciplinary working and the beauty of the arts in hospital when the multi-disciplinary team collaborate.

Listen and watch online 5.2: The Dance Back Home www. artsandhealth.ie/resource/videos/the-dance-back-home/

Language and terminology

The language of science and the humanities are often in stark contrast. Learning to work together is an essential and enriching experience for all involved. Music therapists occupy this shared space through their training and development as clinical professions with a focus on 'treatment', 'clinical outcomes' and 'evidence-based practice'. Community musicians have joined them to a certain extent by adopting terminology such as 'interventions'. Such terminology is controversial to the musicians who claim to work for the artistic benefit only. Whilst the work involved in assessing how music helps, in terms of clinical gains, is valuable and has contributed greatly to specific treatment of symptoms through music, there is also great value in arguing for creativity and beauty in music-making for its own sake rather than for its instrumental benefit. Scientists balk at claims that music will 'make you better' or 'heal you' if not backed up by science. I couldn't agree more, having attended seminars where the central thesis is a belief that music will transform the hospital for the better just by being there. In my work, I found it important to acknowledge the problem of noise pollution from music and the reasons why music might not help someone, in order to build relationships with my colleagues who needed to be able to trust me to be sensible about the role of music in hospital. It is important, also, to recognise that hospital staff bring a wealth of music experiences, talents and resources and can share their music to enrich the environment. Caring for staff through music is important, as well as recognising the many musicians in the team.

Some of the issues currently alive in the field of music in healthcare settings at the current time are discussed below.

Quality and standards of practice

Training and education of musicians is imperative. Currently, music therapists are internationally regulated and must adhere to standards of practice. Musicians, often self-employed and working sessionally, are not required to undergo training or continuous professional development. Standards of practice vary wildly. It is hard to know what best practice is. Professional qualifications, apprenticeships and mentoring or supervision are the building blocks of good practice in all other health professions, so why not for musicians working in healthcare settings? Musicians need to understand basic practice such as confidentiality, professional boundaries, infection control and when to refer a person on to another team member. Standards of practice are subjective and in my experience it can be very difficult to dismiss a musician from the hospital who is under performing (Moss 2007; Moss and O'Neill 2009). Continuing professional development, including mentoring or supervision by an experienced practitioner, is critical to ensuring standards remain high throughout one's career. Self-awareness is also imperative to good practice: for example, knowing what motivates me to engage with people who are ill, awareness of the unconscious processes that drive me to become over involved, and knowing when to step back from engagement or refer a person to other professionals.

Employment issues

Creative artists, such as sessional musicians, self-employed music therapists and composers, are not core healthcare staff and may not get the support they need to work in these environments. Musicians in healthcare benefit from being integrated with the team. Access to clinical supervision, institutional training and employment assistance programmes are essential. Healthcare staff are known to have highly stressful jobs and organisational support is available. Musicians working significant hours in this environment may also need this support.

Lack of funding

Music in healthcare spaces is a contested field where health departments tend to fund only music therapy and arts councils fund only musicians. An anti-therapy bias can exist in arts organisation funding while health settings may focus solely on the instrumental value of the arts. Musicians must navigate these tensions and often find themselves fighting for the crumbs from government health and arts budgets. Limited funding also means that sustaining music practice in healthcare is difficult, and one must continually create exciting pilot projects in order to secure funding. This lack of stability for service users and music and health experts is unsatisfactory, especially where service users have long-term needs or take time to build trusting relationships.

The instrumental and intrinsic value of music

Any aesthetic enrichment undertaken in a hospital must serve a function – to address a clinical need or system problem. Music can serve a functional purpose and does so successfully in many clinical situations. But this is not the whole picture. The inherent value of creativity and its importance in meeting the psychological needs of the whole person needs more recognition. In healthcare spaces, interest often focuses on how music can achieve clinical outcomes – does it reduce blood pressure in people waiting for surgery? Does it relax surgeons in theatre and help them perform better? Does music improve speech post stroke? These are key questions and need to be answered. However, music often plays a different role in society, it has an intrinsic value, not because it achieves a change but because it expresses something universal – it is enjoyable, it is beautiful and/or it brings people together. Gabrielsson's (2011) unique research catalogues the strong experiences people have with music and how music can move us and bond us on a deep level. The evidence in this book complements and arguably goes beyond any scientific theory that explains these experiences. (Gabrielsson 2011; DeNora and Ansdell 2014).

Live vs recorded music

As seen in Chapter 1, recorded music plays an important role in clinical interventions. A pertinent issue of our time is the role of music technology and whether this might replace live music. It is increasingly difficult to argue for the extra cost incurred to provide live music when cheaper technological solutions are available. Evidence throughout this book attests to the importance of the live, relational experience afforded by music-making and performance. Recorded music is a powerful tool, as seen in the care of people with dementia (apps such as Playlist UK offer the opportunity for family and carers to create personally meaningful playlists for people living with dementia). Similarly, recorded music during MRI scanning and other complex procedures can be a powerful distraction from the distress and discomfort of clinical procedures. Future research might do well to focus on how recorded music can best be used, especially for people who cannot control it or make clear choices as to whether they want to listen. However, playlists for people with dementia have been critiqued in terms of lack of control and choice and the potential to isolate people with headphones playing pre-recorded playlists with little human interaction. Technology opens up the possibility of reducing geographical inequality by providing music therapy and music programmes for health online. More research is needed in this area.

Final thoughts

Musicians in healthcare settings are important and must be valued. As a music professional, I recommend engaging and building positive relationships with healthcare staff and clinical teams, trying to meet the needs and difficulties they encounter as a good starting point. It is also important to engage service users in decision making around music in hospital and consider music methods, approaches and interventions that are currently underused in health settings. Flower (2019) writes of the work 'at the edges.' The interesting, most creative work arguably happens at the edges of our practice. As professionals, we need to engage in continuing professional development and be prepared to expand our practice, challenge our assumptions and upskill. We need to engage with music in healthcare spaces as part of the 'interacting contexts' of people, place and things. What is important, and to whom, ebbs and flows as musicking travels across the active edges of hospital performance spaces, music therapy rooms, wards and clinics (Stige 2002; Rolvsjord 2010). Engage only musicians who are flexible and highly qualified to work in your healthcare setting; engage in reflective practice, mentoring and/or supervision yourself to be aware of your own limitations and be cognisant of current health service priorities. Strive for best practice, embrace technology and make links with cultural institutions (Harvey 2018).

Belinda's story

Belinda's story will finish this chapter. Belinda was a woman with profound intellectual disability, caused by childhood illness, and extremely challenging behaviour. She had to be nursed by two nurses at a time due to violence, and when distressed she would smear faeces on the walls. She was doubly incontinent and all personal care routines were stressful and distressing for her. The music therapist who joined the team, Rebecca O'Connor, involved in Belinda's care. The clinical team were at a loss as to how to help her and so they 'tried' music therapy. Gradually, the team became aware that Belinda could occasionally tolerate the guitar playing of the music therapist and would calm down and come out of her room to listen. She began to respond to songs (she could not communicate verbally or understand verbal instruction). The music therapist proceeded to work directly with nurses to address the stressful difficulties they were experiencing in everyday life with Belinda. Together they created songs to signal personal hygiene activities and sessions involved nurses and music therapist in the bathroom with Belinda singing as she brushed her teeth or went to the toilet to enable her to achieve these activities without distress. The music therapist engaged completely with the clinical team and supported both staff and Belinda by addressing real distressful situations in everyday life.

Notes

1 It is important to note that recognition of the clinical profession of Music Therapy varies from country to country, with some having State Registered Professionals (for example UK, USA) but many employing music therapists in the same way as musicians in healthcare (on a contract, sessional, self-employed basis). This creates a natural competition between different music providers for the same pot of funding.
2 Diagram designed by Alison Baker Kerrigan

Further reading

Crawford, P. (2015) *Health humanities*. Basingstoke: Palgrave Macmillan.
Crawford P. and Brown, B. and Charise, A. eds. (2020) *The Routledge companion to health humanities*. Abingdon: Routledge.
DeNora, T. (2013) *Music asylums: well-being through music in everyday life*. Farnham: Ashgate.
Fitzgerald, D. and Callard, F. (2015) *Rethinking interdisciplinarity across the social sciences and neurosciences*. Basingstoke: Palgrave Macmillan.
Rolvsjord, R. (2010) *Resource-oriented music therapy in mental health care*. Gilsum, NH: Barcelona.

References

Ansdell, G. (2014) *How music helps in music therapy and everyday life*. Farnham: Ashgate.
Bonde, L. (2011) Health Musicing – Music Therapy or Music and Health? A Model, Empirical Examples and Personal Reflections. *Music and Arts in Action*, 3(2), 120–40.
Crawford, P. (2015) *Health humanities*. Basingstoke: Palgrave Macmillan.
Crawford P. and Brown, B. and Charise, A. eds. (2020) *The Routledge companion to health humanities*. Abingdon: Routledge.
DeNora T. and Ansdell G. (2014) What can't music do? *Psychology of Well-Being: Theory, Research and Practice* 4, available: http://dx.doi.org/doi:10.1186/s13612-014-0023-6.
Fitzgerald, D. and Callard, F. (2015) *Rethinking interdisciplinarity across the social sciences and neurosciences*. Basingstoke: Palgrave Macmillan.
Fitzpatrick, K., Moss, H. and Harmon, D. (2019) Music in the chronic pain experience: an investigation into the use of music and music therapy by patients and staff at a hospital outpatient pain clinic. *Music and Medicine*, 11, 6–22.
Flower, C. (2019) *Music therapy with children and parents: toward an ecological attitude*. PhD. University of London.

Gabrielsson, A. (2011) *Strong experiences with music*. Oxford: Oxford University Press.

Harvey, A. (2018) *Music, evolution, and the harmony of souls*. Oxford: Oxford University Press.

Levitin, D.J. (2008) *This is your brain on music: understanding a human obsession*. London: Atlantic.

MacDonald, R.A.R. (2013) Music, health, and well-being: a review. *International journal of qualitative studies on health and well-being*, 8, 20635, available: http://dx.doi.org/10.3402/qhw.v8i0.20635.

Moss, H. (2007) Integrating models of music into acute hospitals: an Irish perspective. In Edwards, J., ed., *Music: promoting health and creating community in healthcare contexts*. Newcastle upon Tyne: Cambridge Scholars.

Moss, H. (2016) Arts and health: a new paradigm, *Voices: A World Forum for Music Therapy*, 16(3), available: http://dx.doi.org/doi:10.15845/voices.v16i3.863.

Moss, H., Donnellan, C. and O'Neill, D. (2012) A review of qualitative methodologies used to explore patient perceptions of arts and healthcare. *Medical Humanities*, 38(2), 106–9, available: http://dx.doi.org/10.1136/medhum-2012–010196.

Moss H. and O'Neill D. (2009) What training do artists need to work in healthcare settings? *Medical Humanities*, 35, 101–5, doi: 10.1136/jmh.2009.001792.

Moss, H. and O'Neill, D. (2019) The role of the curator in modern hospitals: a transcontinental perspective. *Journal of Medical Humanities*, 40, 85–100, available: https://doi.org/10.1007/s10912-016-9423-3.

Murphy, L. (2018) The perception of practice of Community Music Therapy in Ireland, *Voices*, 18(2), available: https://doi.org/10.15845/voices.v18i2.947.

Rolvsjord, R. (2010) *Resource-oriented music therapy in mental health care*. Gilsum, NH: Barcelona.

Ross, F. and McSherry, W. (2018) Two questions that ensure person-centred spiritual care, *NursingStandard*, available: https://rcni.com/nursing-standard/features/two-questions-ensure-person-centred-spiritual-care-137261.

Stige, B. (2002) *Culture-centred music therapy*. Gilsum: Barcelona.

Tozer, K. (2015) *What is arts and health?*, available: https://cyhealthcommunications.wordpress.com/2015/11/18/what-is-arts-health/.

Tsiris, G. and Ansdell, G. (2020) Exploring the spiritual in music. *Approaches: An Interdisciplinary Journal of Music Therapy*, 11.

Twyford K. and Watson T. (2008) *Integrated team working music therapy as part of transdisciplinary and collaborative approaches*. London: Jessica Kingsley.

WFMT (2017) *World Federation of Music Therapy*, available: www.wfmt.info.

Final thoughts

As I write the final words of this book, I know that music does matter in hospital, but I also appreciate the questions. Does music cure anyone? Does it reduce bed days or pain medication? Would a person who is in acute abdominal pain really care whether there were musicians or music therapists working in the hospital? In the midst of the Covid-19 pandemic, in which I write the final lines of this book, I see the existence of music in hospital under major threat. Currently, music therapists and musicians across the world are out of work, with hospitals reduced to essential care only, devoid of 'extra' input with many clinical staff struggling to maintain the role and relevance of music in their healthcare setting. Musicians are fighting for survival globally, let alone in hospitals.

There is strong evidence, however, that for some people music makes a concrete difference. For example, the Neurological Music Therapy approach is an evidence-based treatment model that uses standardised, research-based techniques to treat the brain using music and rhythm (Thaut and Homberg 2016). These specific clinical benefits are undisputable. On the other hand, if music is an agent of improved quality of life, aesthetic environment and quality of care, we need to ask if people in hospital really care whether music accompanies them in their hospital journey or as they adapt to living with a chronic illness? This is a significant question, and one many arts practitioners in healthcare do not ask, assuming universal improvement by engaging with the arts.

I am sure, however, from my experience, that music makes a qualitative difference to quality of life and care when used well. I also know that people notice when music is unhelpful, injurious or insensitive in hospital. I am not sure, however, that we can prove, by statistics or quantitative evidence, that quality of care and support matters or makes a difference in hospital settings, let alone the specifics of how music makes such a difference.

Mats' story

During a recent hospital stay in Ireland, when being treated for Covid-19, Mats turned to music to keep his spirits up and to help him feel positive about his recovery chances. Mats is a dance teacher who works in an academy of music and dance with musicians. He listens to music constantly and it is part of his daily life. However, in the strange environment of the hospital ward, with alarms and machines beeping continually, with stress, complete isolation and only meeting tired hospital staff who were dressed in full protective gear, Mats found himself suffering. He describes the environment as not conducive to feeling good. However, WiFi was available, so he took to listening to his favourite musicians on Facebook, who were posting video clips playing his favourite music. He describes lying in bed, physically critically ill, but tapping his feet, dancing in his mind, and enjoying the tunes immensely, thus feeling both peace and strength inside throughout the Covid-19 illness journey. He would also communicate remotely with friends from near and far on how much their music-making meant to him at this time and their replies frequently made him feel even better inside.

Whether or not we prove a beneficial relationship between music and quality of care, it is possible that care and concern about music, art and design reflects a thinking beyond the efficiency and statistics of healthcare, and demonstrates a care and concern for the human receiving care. We will also never find a consensus about what sort of music will 'work' in healthcare, and the only solution I have found is to personalise music to the individual in hospital rather than offer blanket solutions that will irritate some and please others. Personalised, individualised music-making is key – everyone likes different music, everyone has preference for silence, music, background noise, TV or nothing (Moss et al. 2007).

What I do know is that music matters in every society, every age and every culture. Music and creativity are basic human psychological needs and our world is poorer without music (Maslow 1969; Maslow 1970). So if hospital is a microcosm of society, it too needs music. I am compelled by the negative effect of a deficit of music in the hospital environment (aesthetic deprivation) more than by proving the benefit. Without access to music, art and our normal cultural and leisure pursuits, we are likely to do worse, and our psychological well-being will be affected (Maslow 1969; Maslow 1970; Saito 2008; Moss and O'Neill 2014). I also know that during this pandemic, music therapists are still working in hospitals and care homes, playing music from a distance, offering mindful music sessions for stressed caregivers and finding creative ways to work online to offer virtual choirs, playlists and musical care to vulnerable people in healthcare settings.

Jim's story

My first experience as a musician in health and social care was as a volunteer at a day centre for people living with enduring mental health issues, almost thirty years ago. I was an eager, naïve student musician and Jim was a 43-year-old man who had lived for over 20 years with a diagnosis of paranoid schizophrenia. Jim's health issues, heavy medication and illegal drug use had left its toll and he lived with active hallucinations and hearing voices. In those days, side effects of medication were more marked than they are now, and Jim had a significant tremor. His illness manifested itself in poor hygiene, difficulty in talking to others and making social connections and extremely poor concentration. Jim couldn't hold down a job and had little insight into how his drug use and non-compliance with medication affected his health. He trusted few people and was a loner with no regular routine.

The only place and people Jim engaged with were staff and clients at the mental health day centre. However chaotic his lifestyle, the centre offered a place for Jim to visit when he was well enough to engage. He would come and go intermittently, and the staff worried about his health when he didn't show up. He didn't interact much with staff or clients but occasionally engaged in cooking activities or had a meal at the centre. Jim was occasionally verbally aggressive and had damaged property at the centre on two occasions.

As a full-time volunteer, I was asked to engage with the music group on a Wednesday afternoon. This group was an unstructured space where members of the centre played music together. Usually 3–4 members attended. There was no set format, people played together sometimes, other times they just played alone in the same room, sometimes they chatted and worked out how to play a piece together. One staff member played the drums and this sometimes brought coherence to the group as he would facilitate some shared music-making. For a number of weeks I was at the group with Jim. He brought his guitar and I played my trombone. Jim made no eye contact, and had only minimal verbal contact with other members. However, it was immediately clear that Jim was able to connect musically with others in a way that he found extremely difficult verbally.

Jim and I gradually built up a rapport and for a few weeks only the two of us attended the session. Somehow, without talking, we managed to play guitar and trombone together. He was able to play a consistent chord pattern to allow me to improvise a melody with him. He acknowledged me and the music, saying it was good. I noticed he was attending these sessions regularly. What I learned in this, my very first interaction between music and mental health, was to listen and observe. I had no real skills as a music facilitator or therapist. I could play the trombone and had an eagerness to contribute but not a lot else. I attended the music session as a member and a volunteer and watched, learned and listened. There was very little said by anyone at these sessions, very little verbal interaction or negotiation of the music. But we communicated in the music. We tolerated each other's presence and accepted each other through our music-making. I cannot imagine how else I could have built a relationship with Jim except non-verbally, through music. Jim was a homeless, chronically ill, 43-year old man. I was a 22-year-old, middle class, sheltered young woman. It was an unlikely partnership, but it worked. I learned, from listening, about mental health issues, social care issues and the struggles of living with a mental health illness.

I learned four important lessons about music, therapy, health and well-being at the centre. Firstly, no matter how unwell Jim became, the centre staff never gave up on him. There is something crucially important about *staying with people in times of trouble, journeying beside them, no matter what.* Secondly, *no matter how complex our health difficulties, no matter how remote a person is from connecting with others, or how brain damaged, music can reach through and make a connection.* The non-verbal nature of musical communication plays an important part in connecting with people for whom words are difficult. I was hooked on the role music can play in making connections, transforming relationships and bringing hope and beauty to the darkest moments of life. Thirdly, *Jim was aesthetically deprived.* Whilst I had no idea of this concept at the time, it was clear that Jim had no money and could not afford to attend music events. He was too unwell to attend concerts or music festivals. He was unable to commit himself or concentrate long enough to attend a community music group or be a member of a band, and even if he could his personal hygiene and poor social skills would have made this sort of connection very difficult. He had very little awareness of his surroundings or self-care so he could not furnish his home with colour, art or music. He only had his guitar. The Wednesday afternoon music group was his only access to the arts. Since this time I have observed many people I have worked with in healthcare settings who have neglected their arts interests and been deprived by the health care system of their aesthetic and creativity needs. Fourthly, the music session with Jim could only work when it was connected to something bigger, something *interdisciplinary and with the support of a team.*

These four premises have formed the basis of my work as a musician in healthcare settings, a music therapist, a manager, an academic and a teacher of music therapy.

How do we persuade managers, clinicians and senior policy makers that music makes a difference to care? The music therapy community and music experts are together leading research in this area and music is striking ahead of most other art forms, particularly in clinical specialties such as acquired brain injury, autism, palliative care and pain relief. However, it is more difficult, and subtle, to show how music makes a difference in helping people to feel cared for and supported, and the knock on effect of this on compliance to treatment, well-being and positive health outcomes.

This book does not wish to undermine the magnificent work of evidence-based researchers who continue to provide compelling evidence of the benefit of music in specific clinical issues. Music is the artform with the strongest body of high-quality quantitative research regarding health and well-being benefits and I advise readers to study the many references to the systematic reviews in this book. I continue to pursue and present this evidence as part of my work as a researcher of the role of music for health and well-being. However, it is possible that what music can do has been exaggerated and we need a more realistic view of what music can and can't do and how. As eminent writers before me have commented, 'both music and health are more complex, less stable and more emergent than the RCT discourse might allow' (DeNora and Ansdell 2014).

DeNora and Ansdell's evidence from a seven-year ethnographic study bears relevance to me in terms of what music offers in a healthcare environment. Seventeen benefits of music on mental health and well-being *over time* are presented by these authors, including providing a pretext for social relating; providing opportunities for demonstrating skill, receiving praise and bodily movement including dance; doing other things (such as eating and drinking, dressing up, making noise and getting out of the house); providing means for shifting mood, individually and collectively; providing a means for renegotiating one's identity and/or role within group culture or organisation; providing opportunities for interaction with others (and thus opportunities to forge relationships); basic occupation and opportunities for performing/demonstrating success (DeNora and Ansdell 2014).

This book claims that music, properly curated in healthcare spaces, makes a difference to the care of people living with a serious illness and can support staff working in the stressful hospital environment. It contends that we need to listen to service-user stories and that the arts are a particularly effective way to achieve this. Musical narrative is powerful (one only needs to hear a song written for, and performed at, a wedding or funeral to appreciate the power of music to convey emotion, story and intention). We need to be careful about how we programme music in hospital and acknowledge the specialist expertise of the music therapist in this setting. We need to be creative and open to the myriad approaches to music for health and well-being, and to embrace all musical undertaking once it is of a high standard and carefully constructed. We need to seek out excellent examples of music and creativity in healthcare spaces and explore the use music as self-care, whether as a clinician, musician or service user (or all three!)

Finally, I hope this book inspires good practice and an increase in high quality, sensitive music-making in hospitals and improves health and well-being. I also hope it contributes to the valuing of music therapy and music and health practice as something worth investing in, engaging with and centralising within clinical teams.

To conclude I recommend the following:

1. Consult service users regularly and listen to their story.
2. Demonstrate what can be achieved through music, rather than trying to influence through words or explanations.
3. Continually develop your own creativity.
4. Build a core team of staff who appreciate the need for high quality music activities within the hospital.
5. Develop a model or plan for music within the hospital.
6. Explore music for self-care – join a choir, learn an instrument, go to concerts.
7. Create playlists for relaxation, motivation, lifting mood etc. (for yourself and for others!).
8. For relatives or clients with memory loss or cognitive difficulties, create playlists of important music in their life and consider using music to cue important moments in the day (such as bath time or dinner time).
9. Sing! On your own, with colleagues, clients, family and friends.

References

DeNora T. and Ansdell G. (2014) What can't music do? *Psychology of Well-Being: Theory, Research and Practice* 4, available: http://dx.doi.org/doi:10.1186/s13612-014-0023-6.

Maslow, A. (1969) *Toward a psychology of being*. New York: John Wiley & Sons.

Maslow, A. (1970) *Motivation and personality*, 3rd ed. New York: Harper & Row.

Moss, H., Nolan, E. and O'Neill, D. (2007) A cure for the soul? The benefit of live music in the general hospital. *Irish Medical Journal*, 100(10), 636–8.

Moss, H. and O'Neill, D. (2014) The art of medicine: aesthetic deprivation in clinical settings. *The Lancet*, 383(9922), 1032–3, available: http://dx.doi.org/10.1016/S0140-6736(14)60507–9.

Saito, Y. (2008) *Everyday aesthetics*. Oxford: Oxford University Press.

Thaut, M. and Homberg, V. (2016) *Handbook of neurologic music therapy*. Oxford: Oxford University Press.

Index

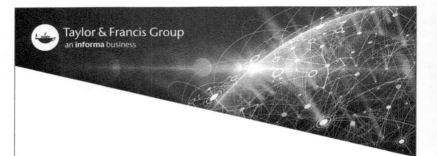

For Product Safety Concerns and Information please contact our EU
representative GPSR@taylorandfrancis.com Taylor & Francis Verlag GmbH,
Kaufingerstraße 24, 80331 München, Germany

Printed and bound by CPI Group (UK) Ltd, Croydon, CR0 4YY
08/06/2025
01896998-0010